Hitchcock's Appetites

Hitchcock's Appetites

The corpulent plots of desire and dread

CASEY MCKITTRICK

Bloomsbury Academic
An imprint of Bloomsbury Publishing Inc

B L O O M S B U R Y
NEW YORK • LONDON • OXFORD • NEW DELHI • SYDNEY

Bloomsbury Academic
An imprint of Bloomsbury Publishing Inc

1385 Broadway
New York
NY 10018
USA

50 Bedford Square
London
WC1B 3DP
UK

www.bloomsbury.com

BLOOMSBURY and the Diana logo are trademarks of Bloomsbury Publishing Plc

First published 2016

Library of Congress Cataloging-in-Publication Data

Names: McKittrick, Casey.
Title: Hitchcock's appetites: the corpulent plots of desire and dread / Casey McKittrick.
Description: New York: Bloomsbury Academic, 2016.
| Includes bibliographical references and index. Identifiers:
LCCN 2015046298 (print) | LCCN 2015047482 (ebook) | ISBN 9781501311659 (hardback)
| ISBN 9781501311628 (epdf) | ISBN 9781501311635 (epub)
Subjects: LCSH: Hitchcock, Alfred, 1899-1980–Health. | Motion picture producers and directors–United States–Biography. | Obesity. | BISAC: PERFORMING ARTS / Individual Director (see also BIOGRAPHY & AUTOBIOGRAPHY / Entertainment & Performing Arts). | PERFORMING ARTS / Film & Video / History & Criticism. Classification: LCC PN1998.3.H58 M45 2016 (print)
| LCC PN1998.3.H58 (ebook) | DDC 791.4302/33092–dc23
LC record available at http://lccn.loc.gov/2015046298

Cover design by Eleanor Rose
Cover image: Still from The Man Who Knew Too Much (1956)
© PARAMOUNT / THE KOBAL COLLECTION

ISBN: HB: 978-1-5013-1165-9
ePDF: 978-1-5013-1162-8
ePub: 978-1-5013-1163-5

Typeset by Deanta Global Publishing Services, Chennai, India
Printed and bound in the United States of America

Contents

Acknowledgments

First, I would like to thank the English Department and the College of Arts and Sciences at Western Michigan University, for their generous support, encouragement, and mentorship. They were instrumental in allowing me to research and write this book, granting me a sabbatical to do archival work and begin the writing process. They were also wonderful listeners and advisors.

I owe the entire first chapter to the fellowship I received in the summer of 2012 from the Harry Ransom Center at the University of Texas at Austin, where I was allowed access to the David O. Selznick and Myron Selznick collections. The help, guidance, and information I received at the Harry Ransom Center made the book a possibility and a fait accompli.

I am deeply indebted, in innumerable ways, to my parents Douglas and Sandra McKittrick, who introduced me to, and let me fall in love with, the films of Alfred Hitchcock.

Janet Staiger has been a constant source of inspiration and support, for having read several of my chapters and shared her own work throughout a career that made me realize productivity and diligence were not just possible, but necessary.

I would probably never have built my own scholarship around the films of Hitchcock if it weren't for a dear friend and mentor, Dr. Sabrina Barton, whose essay on *Strangers on a Train* made me realize that good work in queer and feminist theory could be life-changing and nourishing in profound ways.

The participants of the Hitchcock seminars and the members of the independent study groups at Western, with whom I shared my Hitchcock research, helped me write and grow in ways they will probably never fathom. I owe a debt particularly to Andrea Enyedi, Briana Asmus, and Tazara Owens.

The support I got from friends and colleagues inside and outside the academy made the book happen as well. There are too many to name, but I'd be remiss if I didn't thank John Saillant, Alex Barron, Elizabeth Brenner, Nic Witschi, Meg Dupuis, Kenneth Kidd, Heather Kirksey, Victoria Sheldon Parker, Daryl Kovalich, John Mancuso, Michael Nava, Nicholas Gamble, Christopher Carlsen, Michael Soldier, Steve Berman, Kimberly Hunter Soltero, Pamela Mottley, Shane Dietrich, David Gerstner, Eve Salisbury, Grace Tiffany, Nate Crumpton and other Fourth Coast companions, and Joshua Weaver.

The editors with whom I've worked at Bloomsbury Academic, Katie Gallof and Mary Al-Sayed, have been more than understanding and tolerant of my recent illness, and hearing from them, getting advice from them, has been indispensable to my finishing this project.

Finally, I'd like to thank Neville Hoad and Christopher Nagle for their friendship and their guidance, for providing not just emotional and intellectual support, but also a template of what it means to do scholarship with passion and integrity.

Introduction

They say that inside every fat man is a thin man trying desperately to get out. Now you know that the thin man is the real Alfred Hitchcock.[1]

One sometimes has the impression of Alfred Hitchcock wearing an Alfred Hitchcock mask, or that inside that fat man there is a fat man struggling to get out.[2]

From the time Alfred Hitchcock made his historic 1939 move from Shamley Green, outside London, to Los Angeles to work in Hollywood, until his death forty years later, no publicity piece, film review, or interview with the director was complete without at least a perfunctory reference to, or a loving jab at, his formidable physique. Before he had even acquired that most familiar of monikers, "The Master of Suspense," in 1942, he had been embraced by the American press with headlines like "300-Pound Prophet Comes to Hollywood," "Heavy Heavy . . . Hitchcock," and "Director Hitchcock, Big As An Elephant." A publicity still for his first American picture *Rebecca* reassured us, "'Hitch' doesn't mind allusions to his 239 pounds." Since his passing, the many biographical and critical accounts of the man and his work have continued to find references to his weight, size, or appetites, to be *de rigueur*. Whether these references function as amusing anecdotes about an idiosyncratic auteur, or as more serious and penetrating ruminations on the driving compulsions of his life, they seem to suggest Hitchcock's fatness as a fundamental truth about him.

In some ways, this is a book about the thin man and the fat man identified in the above quotations, and their lifelong attempts to escape from the fleshly prison of a man born Alfred Joseph Hitchcock. It is also about the artist born from this trinity of selves that fought one another for sovereignty of expression. The "mask" described above by Hitchcock biographer John Russell Taylor is that of the globally known and revered persona: the pear-shaped, unflappable, droll, ironic, sweetly morbid Brit who produced fabulous and unpredictable cinema. The thin man trying to escape was an elaborate and important creation of Hitchcock's own mind. He envisioned a man who looked the way he felt: charismatic, limber, romantic, endlessly creative, energetic, and in on the joke. The fat man imagined by Taylor is the one described in Donald Spoto's *The Dark Side of Genius*: a man who hated his body—Hitchcock once called it an "armour of fat"—and even more, hated how his body was read by others, particularly in a culture given to interpret fatness as idleness, stupidity, and lack of self-awareness or discipline. The interplay of these three selves—the public commodity, the ambitious visionary, and the tortured outsider—produced one of cinema's greatest directors, and his greatness, I argue, owes a great deal to his own struggles with the signifying practices of the fat body.

This is the first book-length study of Hitchcock to consider how his experiences as a fat man, and a fat celebrity, found their expression in his cinema.[3] More specifically, the following chapters argue that his fatness informed and inflected his cinematic strategies of representation, his understanding of gender and its embodiment, and, more generally, his conception of the corporeal. They also insist that we cannot understand his relationship to his fatness without also understanding his relationship to food and drink, which were, for him, some of the greatest pleasures in his life, and also the source of his greatest anxieties. Using archival research of Hitchcock's publicity, his script collaborations, and personal communications with producers and media outlets, in tandem with close textual readings of his films, feminist critique, and theories of embodiment, my aim in this book is to produce a new and compelling profile of Hitchcock's creative life, and a fuller, more nuanced account of his auteurism. This profile is an invitation to revisit the Hitchcock oeuvre, with an eye, and a stomach, toward the question of his appetites.

Why appetites?

The question of appetites is likely to crop up, almost implicitly, in any discussion of Alfred Hitchcock and his films. By 1955, the Hitchcock profile was the most recognizable one on the planet, and that may still be the case. In the cultural imaginary, it is difficult, if not impossible, to extract Hitchcock the auteur, the cultural icon, or the historical personage, from his fatness. Nor is it easy to consider Hitchcock apart from his cinematic excesses and the erotics of consumption that permeates his films.

I have named this investigation *Hitchcock's Appetites*, rather than his *Desires* or his *Pleasures*, so as not to invite expectations of a pristinely Lacanian or Barthesian approach. While psychoanalysis and semiotics will prove indispensable to my readings of both Hitchcock and his films in the coming chapters, I have opted for a less disciplinarily saturated term through which to focus my queries. Appetite is an elastic and expansive concept, ensconced in the semiotics of bodily necessity as well as cultural influence and indoctrination. It houses both hunger and taste, imperative and inclination, individual will and powerful predisposition. Appetite is something to be heeded and something to be cultivated; something to be whetted and something to be spoiled. Its Latin origin, *ad* + *petere*, denotes "a seeking to . . ." And the idiom of seeking leads us to many Hitchcockian preoccupations and tropes: compulsion, habit, estrangement, disorientation, misdirection, satiety, lack, and travel.

Appetites, moreover, are semiotically important in that their profession and revelation are intimately bound up in social identity formation. Appetites invariably have indexical value, as they depend upon, and fortify, definitional parameters of gender, race, class, sexuality, and ethnicity. "You are what you eat" may be a glib formulation, though it helpfully gestures to the very human inclination to understand one's profession of tastes as constitutive of character and personality, in culture at large, but also particularly in film narrative. How we perceive professions of taste, and how they align or collide with the values and cognitive codes of the film world, and our own, prescribe how we as spectators come to *know* and assess character. Not only may professions of tastes and appetites reveal the intricacy of filmic personalities to us, but Hitchcock's own professions of tastes—professions often disparate from those he really seemed to embrace—will tell us a great deal about his strategies of self-representation as artist and celebrity.

Appetite appeals to me as an organizing principle as well, particularly in the case of Hitchcock, because of its moral intonations. Bound up in biblical questions of guilt and innocence, appetite appears in Hitchcock's film worlds, either as a symptom or an ultimate determinant of the state of one's very soul. The nature of appetites and whether or not they are heeded, and to what end, are in fact the moral exigencies of biblical narrative, and subsequently the moral stuff of the novel and the feature film. Especially in Hitchcock's world, appetites dictate actions and their consequences. The relationship among appetites, their causes, and effects carves the trajectory of Hitchcockian story and character, never in simple, morally prescriptive ways, but in ways that are certainly value-laden.

Why Hitchcock?

> I am an expert on losing weight. I have lost hundreds of pounds in my lifetime and I represent the survival of the fattest.[4]

> Journalists often ask how much I weigh. I tell them, "Only once a day, before breakfast." The number of pounds, though, must remain a mystery.[5]

Hitchcock was born in Leytonstone, near London, in 1899, just a year and a half before the death of Queen Victoria. As the nineteenth century came to an end, so did the Victorian period and its attendant cultural allowances for male "plumpness," which signified prosperity and good health in a culture marked by poverty and wasting illnesses like tuberculosis. This centennial transition saw several changes in cultural attitudes toward fatness. The social and medical problem of obesity—a category that had remained distinct from the "plump" Victorian gentleman's body—once recognized as a specifically masculine malady, became discursively constructed as a female illness. The fat body, in Britain and especially America, lost its connections to the social elite, and became closely associated with the indeterminately ethnic immigrant and working-class body.[6] Thus, as Hitchcock entered into adulthood in the 1920s, he was cognizant of the social stigma that had begun to visit upon the upwardly mobile fat gentleman. There remained a strong residual Victorian fondness for the figure of portly noblesse, though the encroachment of this new signifying trend threatened to overshadow the more traditional, more permissive views of male fatness.

This cultural shift doubtless influenced Hitchcock's self-perception, instilling class and gender-based anxieties, and these problems only intensified when Hitchcock made his historic move to the more weight-conscious, less forgiving environment of southern California. Hitchcock was plump as a child; he would remark that he had inherited his mother's "cottage loaf" figure, and as he was neither popular nor athletically inclined, his childhood was spent to a large degree alone, save for the companionship of his homemaker mother.[7] In speaking with his family friend Charlotte Chandler, Hitchcock wistfully evoked the evanescent Victorian mentality about maleness and size, this time in the context of childhood. He mused, "Plumpness in very small children was considered 'cute' and even a sign of good health. It reflected well on the parents and their prosperity, and showed they were taking good care of their child."[8] As he grew into adulthood, his five-foot six-inch frame already supported a greater weight than was thought healthy by conventional medicine. Over the next fifty years, his weight would fluctuate drastically and often, dipping briefly down to 189 pounds at its lowest, usually registering over 250, and occasionally creeping up to what was medically considered a dangerous 300 pounds.

Hitchcock, who self-reports that he had never had a drop of liquor before he was twenty-four years old, confided to American reporters in 1937, "I first started to put on weight when I took to drink."[9] The director certainly struggled with regulating his intake of both food and alcohol throughout his adulthood. By the time he moved to Hollywood in 1939 to make *Rebecca* for Selznick International Pictures, his weight for the first time had threatened to reach the 300-pound mark. At this time, he was also drinking quite heavily, enjoying pitchers of gin and orange juice with writers and other collaborators, and consuming a pint or two of champagne at lunch before the afternoon shoots, through which he would often slumber. His reputation as a lush who would fall asleep in public was born in Hollywood in his first few years there, and persisted even in the stretches of his abstention from drink in the mid-1940s and early 1950s.

The death in 1942 of Hitchcock's mother and, shortly after, his brother, galvanized Hitchcock for the first time to adopt a serious and successful, if impermanent, plan of weight loss.[10] He began dieting during the making of *Shadow of a Doubt* (1943), and by the end of production on *Lifeboat* (1944), he was able to show off a nearly-100-pound weight loss in a photo cameo in the film, which showed him in a fictitious Before and After campaign for Reduco, a diet pill. His weight fluctuated greatly for the next ten years. Hitchcock was at his trimmest during his Golden Age of filmmaking (189 pounds during 1954's *Rear Window*, and closer to 200 for the next six years, carrying him through *The Man Who Knew Too Much*, *Vertigo*, *North By Northwest*, and *Psycho*). For the remainder of the 1960s and 1970s, his weight slowly returned to nearly 300 pounds, until his death in 1980.

Hitchcock had a great passion for fine food and quality wine and liquor. At great expense, he had Dover sole, beef, and lamb flown in weekly from England, and paté de foie gras from Maxim's in Paris. The only major renovations on his and his wife's (Alma) modest home—they had bought it for 40,000 dollars—in Los Angeles came in the form of a new wine cellar and a bigger kitchen (their favorite room in the house) with additional cold storage. In 1960, Hitchcock became Chevalier du Tastevin in Dijon, France, an order of wine connoisseurs that qualified him as an expert.[11] He would occasionally drink liquor during working hours, though for many years he claimed to wait until 5:00 p.m. to partake. He often enjoyed a drink before dinner: mimosas, gin and orange juice, a tumbler of Cointreau. He and Alma served wine every night at dinner, often a Pouilly Fuisse, a Musigny, a Vin Gris, or Montrachet. Brandy was usually poured after dessert, which could be strawberries and cream, an English trifle, blackberry pie, or a cold fruit mousse.[12]

The Hitchcocks dined out often on Thursday nights, frequently at Chasen's in West Hollywood, which Hitchcock patronized for its refusal to cave in to new trends in lighter, healthier restaurant fare. Raised on hearty recipes containing suet, leaf lard, and dripping, he detested the substitution of light seed and vegetable oils in the preparation of his favorite dishes. A typical dinner at home, for the couple alone, would consist of a boiled ham and roasted chicken, new potatoes, rolls, a salad, and a dessert. Their daughter Patricia recalls a visiting friend who saw Alma preparing dinner and asked, "How many people are you expecting tonight?" The guest was nonplussed by her casual reply, "Just the two of us."[13]

The couple hosted weekend guests with some regularity and threw dinner parties for their colleagues. Hitch and Alma prepared every detail of the meals well in advance, consulting with their cook (when they had one; Alma did most of the cooking, and Hitchcock would occasionally help clean up). What follows is the menu plan Alma drafted for a weekend at their second home in Santa Cruz, April 12–14, 1963, where the couple entertained writer Joan Harrison and her husband, and writer, Samuel Taylor:

Friday, Dinner:
Spinach soup
Santa Cruz fish
Allumette potatoes
Artichokes
Pears Helene

Saturday, Lunch:
Melon
Irish ham with Madeira sauce
Puree of peas
Pommes puree
Strawberries, crème double

Saturday, Dinner:
Paté Maison (with cocktails)
Roast ducks
Apple sauce, peas, new potatoes
"Pickwick" ice pudding
Coffee

Sunday Brunch:
Grapefruit
Mixed grill: bacon, sausages,
kidneys, tomatoes, mushrooms,
Popovers
Pineapple

Sunday Dinner:
English Turbot, hollandaise sauce
Saddle of lamb
Asparagus, roast potatoes
Vanilla ring with peaches, raspberry sauce
Coffee, liquors

In his life and in his cinema, Hitchcock clearly expressed the centrality of food and drink to his quest for the good life. He engaged in constant metaphorical play with concepts of food, hunger, consumption, curiosity, and knowledge. He enjoyed the evocative parallels between visual and gustatory pleasure, and understood audiences' appetites as encompassing both the corporeal and the cerebral. In exemplary fashion, he made rhetorical inversions such as his famous, "Man does not live by murder alone. He needs affection, approval, encouragement and, occasionally, a hearty meal." In "Conversation Over a Corpse," an episode of his television show, he offers, "As you may know, food is a hobby of mine. I don't claim to be an expert cook, but I am rather a good eater. If you will wander into my kitchen, I'll allow you to watch me as I concoct some delicacy to tempt your palate." Time and again, on Hitchcock's screen, mise-en-place begets mise-en-scene. Murder is staged for the spectator in culinary terms, an event in itself, to be consumed and relished. The playful analogies—the back and forth of food and crime, of meat and plotting—served the director well. The Hitchcockian cinematic aesthetic relies on troping hunger—culinary, libidinal, narrative—to *produce* and *satisfy* hunger in his audiences. He famously quipped, "For me, the cinema is not a slice of life, but a piece of cake." Not cross-section, but confection; not microcosm, but meal; his cinematic offering was the gift of visual and visceral pleasure. These very pleasures he himself enjoyed, however, carried disillusioning consequences, and his body became an expression of both pleasure and its regret.

Hitchcock studies and fat studies: An interdisciplinary repulsion?

As I have mentioned, Hitchcock scholarship has chiefly focused on the director's weight and size only to the extent that it provides anecdotal amusement, a superficial understanding of his idiosyncrasy, or an allusion to the "dark" forces of resentment and self-loathing at work beneath the surface. That his own embodied experience may be an important interpretive lens through which to view his art has rarely been broached. Equally puzzling (to this critic) is the virtual absence of even a mention of Hitchcock in the corpus of available fat studies scholarship. Alongside William Howard Taft, Winston Churchill, Roscoe "Fatty" Arbuckle, Luciano Pavarotti, and Diego Rivera, Hitchcock is one of the more culturally, and perhaps historically, important fat men of the twentieth century. So how does one account for what is either apathy or resistance to exploring the role fatness played in the life, the art, and the cultural reception of one of the world's most famous directors?

In their introduction to a pioneering anthology, *The Fat Studies Reader*, editors Esther Rothblum and Sondra Solovay situate their emerging discipline thusly:

> In the tradition of critical race studies, queer studies, and women's studies, fat studies is an interdisciplinary field of scholarship marked by an aggressive, consistent, rigorous critique of the negative assumptions, stereotypes and stigma placed on fat and the fat body.

Rothblum and Solovay ground the definition of their field in references to academic studies of race, gender, and sexuality, because, like fat studies, each discipline had its roots in social activism that sought to end oppression based on a marginalized identity and body, and thus, its later development within the academy was organized around bodily difference and disenfranchisement. The often unhappy marriage of academia with disciplines founded on contested identity politics has been further complicated in the case of fat studies, in part because, like LGBT studies in its early days (and to some degree, still), it has been perceived by some as espousing a rhetoric of victimization and coercion that is incommensurate with the "common sense" notion that being fat (like being gay) is a choice. Thus arises a kind of false dichotomy, between an essentialist body politics of race and gender, and a superfluous or indulgent body politics of fatness (and/or queerness). Unfortunately, the destructive and degrading cultural paradigms that equate fatness with ignorance, vice, and lack of discipline—the very paradigms fat studies scholars seek to challenge—operate in the academy to question and often discount the legitimacy of the field as intellectually viable.

Not only is fat studies a nascent academic discipline that has been met with a degree of institutional resistance, but its central object of analysis—fat—presents theoretical difficulties in the diffuse and staggering versatility of its denotative and connotative possibilities. We can approach fat through various points of entry, alternately considering it as:

- a medical condition
- an aesthetic or cosmetic problem

- a politicized identity
- a private or personal experience
- a commodity
- a symptom of personality or temperament
- a social problem
- an erotic feature or fetish
- a hereditary burden
- a record of consumption
- a stigma or taboo
- a shield or buffer
- a blatant or intrusive presence

Clearly, to understand fat in all of its social, medical, legal, rhetorical, aesthetic, and physical dimensions requires focused and committed contributions from disciplines as diverse as anthropology, sociology, medicine, literary studies, economics, law, women's studies, and many more. Otherwise fat studies, isolated from more established and sanctioned disciplines, will continue to be marginalized in curriculum and ghettoized in the embattled "_______ Studies" model.

Another reason that Hitchcock studies and fat studies may mutually resist productive exchange is the entrenched and somewhat erroneous perception of fat studies as a discipline predominantly oriented toward females, both as practitioners and subjects of analysis. In his book *Fat Boys*, which examines the meanings and the status of American fat masculinity in the twentieth century, Sander Gilman expresses a frustration with the relative exclusion of men from the scholarship, not to mention the activism, of fat studies. He proclaims:

> Over and over again the issue of size and the issue of diet have been seen as primarily of concern to *women*. There have been very few detailed studies of the complex history of the relationship between *men* and fat because of the assumption that fat is purely a feminist issue.

Gilman's desire for more studies that include men and the male body in the histories and theories of fat is understandable and shared by this writer, though the "purely" in his formulation is a bit troublesome for me. The often heard mantra "Fat is a feminist issue" effectively draws attention to the notion that women are oppressed through the unrealistic, constraining, patriarchally sanctioned definitions of normative female body size and size-based standards of beauty that circulate in Western culture.

However, when Gilman questions "the assumption that fat is purely a feminist issue," I hear a conflation of feminism and woman, with the unsettling reverberation that only women are the subjects of feminist analysis or social activism. Feminism rightfully proceeds from a premier commitment to women, their bodies, their safety, and their equality. Yet, as an academic discipline, the theorization of masculinity, fat and otherwise, is necessary to understand gender as an ideological category and a matrix of hierarchized lived experience. Thus, when Gilman suggests that fat is "more than" a feminist issue, I assume either that he means to say "more than a woman's issue," or that he sees the fat male body as somehow outside the purview of feminist analysis. And I am hard-pressed to think of a feminist critique of embodiment that ignores the differences between how male and female bodies are interpreted, and consequently treated, in a given cultural setting. That being said, the perception of fat studies as a female-centered discipline is widely shared in and outside academia.

If we look more specifically at the case of Hitchcock studies, the gender of disciplinary language and disciplinarity itself may be at issue in accounting for its disconnection from fat studies. Obviously, Hitchcock as an artist and historical personage has been more often the subject of humanities scholarship than the social sciences. While fat studies certainly has usefulness in literary interpretation, and humanities scholars have evoked the questions and frameworks of fat studies to perform their own analyses, by and large the field consists of the social scientific contributions of anthropology, sociology, and women's studies. As a frequent subject of humanities work, Hitchcock is often portrayed in the idiom of genius, of transcendence, and inspiration, and these concepts have markedly less purchase in the discourses of social sciences, which tend to value the language of empiricism and quantitative measurement (though certainly there are exceptions).

If fat studies is invested in understanding the mechanisms by which fat people suffer at the hands of prejudicial, fat-phobic social policies, toxic environments, and internalized standards of beauty and acceptability, it follows that its subjects of analysis are inevitably described as marginalized by such practices and sentiments. Hitchcock may have found no traction (so far) in fat studies because, from a materialist perspective, he is far from a socially or economically marginal figure. Hitchcock's body encapsulated two strong and strongly contradictory sets of signifiers. One, that of the looming, bulging patriarch, the "fat cat" (notice the positive masculine connotations of "fat" here) with abundant resources—both material and human—at his disposal. The other, of the unhealthy, unattractive, and culturally abject spectacle associated with obesity. On one hand, Hitchcock was among the wealthiest directors in Hollywood by the time he had struck a television deal for his *Alfred Hitchcock Presents* in the mid-1950s. At the top of his career, he had the attentions and the virtual carte blanche of Warner Brothers, Paramount, and Universal Studios. He had a solid companionate marriage, a healthy, successful child, and several homes that served as sanctuary and seat of society. Actors lined up to work with him, and global audiences lined up for his latest production. On the other hand, all of these kudos and acquisitions could not lessen the feelings of loss and shame he harbored around the embarrassment of his body, and thus, his manhood. These polarized meanings—the very powerful and the powerless—contended with one another for dominance throughout Hitchcock's life and career. A synthesis of the two was impossible, so the story of the Master of Suspense is a story of the swift and unpredictable vacillation between these radically different social, psychological, and rhetorical positions.

These vexed signifiers become even more discordant in their intermingling with the gendered discourse of Hitchcock's purported genius. I would venture further to suggest that the language of the genius and of the transcendent artist is a predominantly masculine one (and I am moved to, but hesitant to, call it patriarchal). For example, William Rothman, in his *Hitchcock: The Murderous Gaze*, refers to the director as having "godlike powers" and describes the compulsion of even the "blindest viewer to bow before the terrifying power his camera commands."[14] This discourse of mastery seems strangely out of line with the more feminized discourse of self-esteem that operates within fat studies, in its interrogation of the psychological trauma that fat oppression gives rise to. The semiotics of the genius or the quintessential artist carries with it the notion of profound self-actualization, and thus, in this vein of humanities writing, to place an artist like Hitchcock within a disciplinary framework that privileges both political correctness and the language of psychic vulnerability and self-worth is either to place a fish on a bicycle, or to trivialize the artist's greatness. In other words, the Hitchcock of many literary accounts is presumed to be exempt from the contingencies of social theories—especially ones that see him as potentially marginal.

Despite their differences in disciplinary orientation and the seeming incompatibility of the gendered language that governs them, I firmly believe that, in the case of Hitchcock, the critical approaches of fat studies only enhance and illuminate understandings of the director, both in his public and professional life, and in his cinematic productions. This book represents a concerted effort to bridge the disciplines of fat studies and Hitchcock studies so that each may speak productively to the other. I am hopeful, and confident, that this study produces more interdisciplinary insight than disciplinary cross-contamination.

Hitchcock, feminism, and embodiment

One of the founding assumptions of this book is that a fat studies approach necessarily entails a feminist commitment and sensibility. As a child, my father introduced me to the pleasures of Hitchcock, and in my formal education, Hitchcock ensnared me via a bracing, life-changing graduate seminar, Feminist Film Theory, conducted by film scholar Dr. Sabrina Barton. As a gay man raised and nourished lovingly, if strictly, by the feminism of Judith Butler, Teresa de Lauretis et al., and prompted to fundamentally recalibrate my notions of desire and identity by the queer theory of Eve Sedgwick, Gayle Rubin, and Lee Edelman, I have had an ongoing strong, often frustrating, investment in reconciling my love for Hitchcock's cinema with a politics of gender and sexuality I can live with. Even as a man, I identify as one of "Hitchcock's daughters," a name Tania Modleski gives to the female spectator who recognizes the deeply problematic nature of Hitchcock's often degrading representations of women, and the narrative economy which uses female suffering as the fuel for the machinery of narrative pleasure, but at the same time, remains committed to mining his films' less obvious pleasures, which come from discerning moments of female patriarchal resistance and the undoing of patriarchal logic.

Modleski argues, in her *The Women Who Knew Too Much: Hitchcock and Feminist Theory*, that a fundamental ambivalence characterizes Hitchcock's relationship with femininity.[15] Her study builds a model of spectatorship that counters (or at least complicates) Laura Mulvey's initial claims in "Visual Pleasure and Narrative Cinema" that the cinematic apparatus's deployment of the male gaze (with Hitchcock as exemplum) leaves the female viewer with the sole option of masochistic identification.[16] Claiming "*neither* that Hitchcock is utterly misogynistic *nor* that he is largely sympathetic to women and their plight in patriarchy," she sketches an ambivalence that manifests itself as "a strong fascination and identification with [cinematic] femininity [that] subverts the claims to mastery and authority not only of the male characters but of the director himself."[17]

I too am invested in eschewing a picture of Hitchcock that takes his films as fundamentally misogynist or radically progressive in a feminist vein. And like Modleski, I believe that ambivalence is the most illuminating and rewarding way to characterize Hitchcock's consideration of cinematic femininity. In this book, I chart a slightly different set of ambivalent directorial feelings—a set that may be seen as a corollary to Modleski's, though not necessarily. The ambivalence I mean to elucidate as part of this book's project is rooted in Hitchcock's experience of fat embodiment, less determined by and determining *of* psychoanalytic processes, though equally attuned to issues of desire and identification.

Hitchcock understood cinematic femininity, just as he understood cultural femininity, to be an elaborate fiction, having little to do with an essential womanhood and more to do with patriarchal fantasy. What is more, he appreciated women as cultural hard workers, who strived to perform this version of femininity as spectacle intended for male consumption. Hitchcock himself possessed all the self-consciousness and vulnerability of one who experiences this double consciousness, who was aware of his own status as visual spectacle despite his privileged position as a wealthy white heterosexual man and as a cinematic creator who deployed such spectacle himself. He understood that, much like women, he was read first and indelibly by the contours of his body and by the cultural paradigms that ascribed value to his fatness. His awareness of the arbitrary nature of female signification, however, did not necessarily yield a competence for gleaning the extent to which women suffered unjustly for these coerced performances.

At the same time, Hitchcock often perceived his obesity as a threat to his masculinity; the feminizing properties of fat—its connotations of the "soft," "yielding," "pliant," "frivolous," "superfluous," "weak," and "malleable"—rendered it a devastating source of shame, resulting in a hostile, contemptuous, compensatory need to disavow his affinities with and connections to the feminine. Thus, we may read the precarity, suffering, and murder of women in his films as symbolic erasures of the dangerous feminine which had to be purged to shore up the lines of his own masculinity.

This second description of Hitchcock's relationship with femininity via the vicissitudes of his embodied experience as a fat man does not exempt him from allegations of misogynist attitudes nor from interpretations of his cinema that find misogynist representations of women. In fact, my description of this version of Hitchcockian ambivalence might strike some as the very textbook case of misogyny. These tendencies to scapegoat women, however, must be considered alongside the mitigating humanizing, empathetic impulses that his shared double-consciousness allowed him toward women. For him, coercive ideologies, the physical and cultural "truths" of embodiment—not women—were the true enemy, even if his cinema demonstrates that he was not always able to differentiate between the dancer and the dance.

How Hitchcock's body matters

As a professor of film, when I introduce my students to auteur theory, or even just directorial style, I start by addressing the paradox of authorship in the context of a highly collaborative medium like film. If a single unifying voice or vision can be expressed in the medium, I tell them, we may find it through the enunciation of a particular worldview, a distinguishing motif, a recurring set of concerns, a go-to camera set up, a lingering theme, or some assemblage of these traits. Directorial style, which Hitchcock cleverly defined as "self-plagiarism," is the authorial signature on a film, I used to explain in my lecture. Nowadays, I am more inclined to liken style to an authorial thumbprint. Often, the class will debate which is the more apt metaphor for directorial style—the autograph or the fingerprint—(and if I am feeling energetic or ambitious, I offer as alternative imprinting images the "snow angel," the "breath on glass," the "right hook," the "lipstick trace," the hickey.) All in all, I am most drawn to the image of the thumbprint for admittedly essentialist reasons: I like the notion of the director's imprinting a record of her anatomical uniqueness onto her filmic creation.

This image of the thumbprint appeals to me, I believe, mostly because it foregrounds the importance of the director's own embodiment (and perception of it) as formative and essential in the creative process. In recent years, stunning scholarship has emerged interrogating the role of sensation and embodiment in the cinematic spectator, and how sensory experience feeds into the affective and cognitive dimensions of how we watch and interpret films. Work by scholars as diverse as Janet Staiger, Vivian Sobchack, Steven Shaviro, and Linda Williams, informed by earlier work on the body and pleasure by the likes of Gilles Deleuze and Felix Guattari, Roland Barthes, and Christian Metz, have insisted productively on the recognition of the embodied spectator. Yet, whereas it is quite easy, empirically speaking, to measure the ways that cinema acts on bodies—there, in the theater, on the sofa, at the computer desk, we can record the presence of chills, tears, screams, yawns, snores, as a film unfolds—accounting for the ways that (directors') bodies act on their cinematic productions is mostly speculative, anecdotal, and uncomfortably abstract.

Yet, as a theorist of film and the body, and a writer who has more than occasionally experienced life as a fat man, I have an aversion to romantic notions of the disembodied genius, artist, or storyteller, and for that reason, I am committed to the notion that Hitchcock's weight, his size, and his experience of fatness were never incidental to his art. For the figures at *both* ends of the camera, films are embodied performances of empathy, otherness, mimesis, kinetic worlding, gender traversing, and existential forensics. Movies contain the echo, the trace, the stain, the genetic code, what have you, of their creators. One of my central goals in this book is to direct attention to the ways that Hitchcock's embodiment speaks through his films and through records of his public life.

Chapter 1, "Hitchcock's Hollywood Diet" tells a new story of Hitchcock's first ten years in the United States, revisiting his professional relationship with

David O. Selznick. The producer and director together engaged in an intensive publicity campaign to establish the Master of Suspense as one of Europe's greatest cinematic exports, and to build the sensational profile that eventually consolidated into the Hitchcock brand, they employed the spectacle of his fatness to generate a unique and potent image. The commodification of Hitchcock's size, however, was exploited in more insidious ways as well. Selznick and his cronies often used Hitchcock's weight as a means of shaming him into silence or equivocation, regarding the demands he made concerning his salary, his choice of projects, his production schedule, and other business aspirations. In short, Hitchcock's early Hollywood career was profoundly affected by the manipulation, both well-intentioned and malignant, of anxieties about his fat body.

Hitchcock's illustrious film career proceeded alongside ever-evolving regimens of dieting, of weight fluctuation, of abstention from food and drink, and of disappointing surrender to his favorite pleasures. Although Hitchcock had a strong exhibitionist streak—he once claimed to have "the heart of a performer"—and enjoyed performing in many different capacities, his size and shape precluded the possibilities of his cinematic stardom. The fact of his fatness alienated him from the very economy of romance and desire that structured his own cinema, and while he publicly disparaged actors as needy and narcissistic, and downplayed the importance of actorly craft, his exclusion from this economy of desire was a private source of angst. Chapter 2, "The Hitchcock Cameo: Fat Self-Fashioning and Cinematic Belonging," examines the cameo appearances in his motion pictures as a compromise between his desire for visibility and attention, and the cinematic codes of acceptable masculinity that checked these desires. The cameo, originating in his 1927 *The Lodger* and recurring all the way up to his final film *Family Plot* in 1976, was a ritual that performed several symbolic gestures. First, it served as a reminder of and homage to his early days of filmmaking in Britain when modest and intimate productions made his participation in the films "necessary," and thus, became a ritual that bridged his early ensemble productions with his later Hollywood efforts which were high-budget, populated by a cast and crew of hundreds, if not thousands, and characterized by high commercial expectations.

Second, it functioned as a sort of authorial signature, whereby he could insert himself in a mode I term *mesogetic*—a narrative mode that lies within the film's diegesis, but which effects a straining, not quite puncturing, intrusion from the extra-diegetic, and allowing their intertextual interplay. Third, the long-lived ritual of the cameo enacted a conferral of cinematic belonging, whereby Hitchcock could see himself as being *of* the screen, not just the orchestrator behind it; the appearances he made constituted proof of his body's *cinematicity*, and this sense of cinematic belonging soothed his sense of exclusion from the ranks of stardom.

Chapter 3, "The Pleasures and Pangs of Hitchcockian Consumption," investigates the various ways Hitchcock employed his greatest pleasures—food and drink—in the service of cinematic visual and narrative pleasure. At the same time, it probes his deployment of images of consumption and elimination to evoke strong experiences of *displeasure*, dis-identification, and nausea. For Hitchcock, attention to the minutiae of food and drink in his filmmaking was part and parcel of his dogged commitment to verisimilitude, to the construction of a mise-en-scene that represented a rich and authentic understanding of place and time. Apart from his deployment of food and drink as a practice of his realist aesthetic, he also portrayed consumption of food and drink as moments that evinced philosophical inquiry into the relationship between pleasure and disgust—a duality arising from his own habits of consumption that never found resolution in his lifetime. Food and drink become reliable indices of character in many instances of Hitchcock's filmmaking; his creations become knowable through what they hold dear and what makes them weak. Food in particular functions to dramatize sublimation, vulnerability, and ambivalence; it metaphorizes the narrative flow of information and the nature of his characters' interactions. Above all, Hitchcock employed food as part of a triad of visual and narrative pleasure, alongside sex and murder, to explore how these pleasures constitute one another, metaphorically and metonymically. These pleasures, however fleeting or at times unattainable, ground the motives and meanings of the characters that populate his film world.

Chapter 4, "Appetite and Temporality in *Rear Window*: Another Aspect of Voyeurism," offers insight into one of the most successful films of Hitchcock's Golden Age. The many pressures, encouragements, and, above all, frustrations, wrought by his struggle with food and drink fed the director creatively; his meditations on the nature of size, growth, change, and desire find truly provocative and variegated expression in the story world of L. B. Jeffries—one that has until now been explicated predominantly in terms of its meta-cinematic qualities and its exploration of desire and objectification's connection to the male gaze. In addition to the film being a stunning visual meta-cinematic essay, a meditation on the active and passive, subjective and objective, exploitative and ethical facets of the gaze, it is also an intervention into the gaze as purveyor of the fantasy of the scopic object's fixity. This false notion of the atemporality of the object of the gaze, this misunderstanding of the erotic object's being forever frozen in or outside of time, which follows from the complementary fantasy of mastery and control conferred on the desiring subject, must be recognized by Jeffries before he can consent to the romantic propositions that Lisa Freemont has extended. Thus, a crucial part of Jeffries's adoption of the ethical, humanizing gaze is the recognition of the woman as dynamic, subject to time and change, and human. The film's visual tropes of size, growth, proportion, and change engage and subvert the cinematic apparatus as guarantor of mastery and fetishistic distance.

Chapter 5, "Children and the Challenge of Fat Masculinity," returns us to a probing of how Hitchcock's vulnerability around his weight and his own habits of consumption led to certain debilitating anxieties about his manhood. One way in which he kept these anxieties in check was to police very carefully the public perception of his masculinity, which for him meant the repeated and pronounced disavowal of sentimentality, maternity, and other feminine significations. His famous dislike for eggs and pregnant women, long a part of the public circulation of Hitchcockian lore, may not be simple markers of endearing idiosyncrasy and taste, but attempted correctives to the cultural paradigms that link the fat male body to effeminacy, maternity, and emotional susceptibility. The anti-child humor that punctuated his public appearances in print and frame, coupled with the choices he made in cinematic representations of childhood—as absent, under attack, traumatic, or antagonistic—reveal the intentional construction of an image of the director that is starkly unsentimental and gruff, which departs dramatically from the impression of those close to him who report his warmth and fondness for children. While this manipulation of public image may have just as much to do with Hitchcock's desire to dis-identify with the bourgeois homogeneity of the American middle class, the director's resolve to keep a "masculine atmosphere" in his filmmaking foregrounds his concerns about how his fatness and gender performance may implicate one another in undesirable ways.

Chapter 6, "Hitchcock and the Queer Lens of Fatness," situates the director in the context of the overlapping discourses of Queer Theory and Fat Studies. The recent work of body theorists has produced the insight that fatness as a category queers the body, in its destabilizing challenge to what constitutes the "normal," "natural," "healthy," and "historical" state of the human body. The fat body is transgressive, with corporeal boundaries that confound the prescriptions of normative signification. Hitchcock's fraught relation to the normative body provides a starting point for a discussion of the queerness of not simply his body, but his own senses of desire and identification, both as he expressed them cinematically and in his interpersonal relationships. To argue for Hitchcock's queerness is not to suggest that he was homosexual, either in his sexual practices or in his self-perception, nor is it to exonerate him from allegations of homophobia and misogyny on many fronts. Rather, understanding the queer nature of Hitchcock and his cinema in particular is to exempt him from formulaic accounts of cinematic processes of desire and identification that traditionally have underwritten the project of a coercive heterosexual reproductive futurism. Far from orchestrating a tight and discretely segmented apparatus of the active male gaze and passive female object, Hitchcock reveals the workings of fantasy as modes of imaginative engagement that refuse to rely on prescriptive gendered ways of looking. Romantic heterosexuality in his cinema is always of suspect origin, motivation, and shelf life. In his cynical layering of traditional romantic desire with perversities and caveats of normativity, he is importantly resistant to the easy and genial futurism that operates eschatologically for many of his director peers in the Classical Hollywood Cinema. These queer spins on the dynamics of cinematic desire were enabled by the vantage points afforded by Hitchcock's exclusion from normative modes of love and romance.

The genius of tall, thin, and handsome

One of my favorite quotations from Hitchcock is a lesser known one that I came across while researching for this book. He once told Charlotte Chandler, "I never achieved the body I wanted, though I am proud of my body of work. It is tall and thin and handsome." It is a clever play on body and corpus, of course, but it is also incredibly poignant and profoundly relevant to this study. The chapters herein represent rudimentary attempts to analyze his film texts and re-narrate pieces of the Hitchcock biography through this lens of his embodied fat experience. I hope that this new perspective on the director may excite scholars and critics into adding to, and complicating, the ideas born out of the encounter between Hitchcock and fat studies.

In the pages to come, I address how Hitchcock's body affected the course of his career, how he commodified his fat to achieve fame and great wealth, how fat was used to manipulate him into making certain career choices, why his cameo appearances mattered to him, how food and drink were employed by the artist to make commentary on both character and consumption, and how fatness shaped his understanding of gender and desire. One thing I have barely broached is my earlier, perhaps puzzling, contention that Hitchcock's fatness is tied to his genius. Though I have commented on the tendencies for humanities scholars to describe the Master of Suspense using the language of genius, with its attendant rhetoric—timelessness, transcendence, universalism—as a scholar, I have a hard time leaving the concept of the genius alone.

I am very clearly indebted, in this book, to the biographical scholarship of John Russell Taylor, who produced the authorized biography *Hitch: The Life and Times of Alfred Hitchcock*, Donald Spoto, the scribe of *The Dark Side of Genius: The Life of Alfred Hitchcock*, and Patrick McGilligan, who offers the cogent, lucid, inspired account of Hitch in *Alfred Hitchcock: A Life in Darkness and Light*. I could not have written this account of the director without their rigor, insight, and industriousness. Yet I feel the need to nitpick for a moment, in order to address this question of fatness and genius.

When I read Spoto's biography, I am always moved and impressed by the depth and breadth of his meticulous collection of biographical data, anecdotes, his rich swatches of Hollywood history. At the same time, my reading is tempered and somewhat tainted in that I feel far too often as if I am reading a melodrama. And this is not a knee-jerk response to a first-time engagement with the book. Read after read, I register the same complaint: *He deserves better.* No, I am not looking for exoneration from or rationalization of his bad behavior, but I am looking for a more humanizing approach that this language of the "dark side" and "genius" do not seem to permit.

This book is a project of humanization much more so than it is one of canonization. It is also an interrogation of genius. As a scholar I distrust the word "genius," and yet I feel I am in the presence of one each time I start a Hitchcock film. I am always looking to resolve this personal contradiction, and after starting this book, I realized that Hitchcock's fatness may be one point of entry into this fraught conception of artistic transcendence. My inclination is to demystify the notion of "genius" by seeing it as alternative, largely untapped emotional and critical resources that mobilize or surface in response to trauma or depressive influence. And Hitchcock's experience of fatness, complicated by the reactions of peers, publics, and intimates to his appetites and his size, martialed these exceptional, little used frameworks for looking at life, love, physicality, and representation differently, and more expansively.

As I have said, Hitchcock hated his body and even more so, hated the way his body was read. He hated the cultural associations of fatness with lethargy, stupidity, dullness, commonness, and I argue that what we call "genius" is actually Hitchcock's passionate, lifelong attempt to prove his many, many *leannesses*. He was desperate that the world should know the "thin man" within, and that his fat exterior (and his troubles with food and drink) was the exception to, not the rule of, his character. These compensatory attempts to be seen for the man he felt himself to become in so many forms, ranging from his daily dressing to the nines in immaculate suits, to his insistence on tight shots over wide ones, to his incredibly conservative attitude toward the use of revealing long shots, to his concept of "pictorial tension," to his having one of the smallest ratios of shot footage to printed footage in Hollywood history. He constantly tried to prove that he was not wasteful, that he was resourceful, mindful of detail, that his filmmaking was disciplined, tight, taut, compact, muscular—everything his body was not. He saw his art in terms of metaphors of the body, and sought to transform people's views of his body through the constant display of innovation (he hated clichés, because he hated "obviousness," another signifier of the fat body), judiciousness (never an inch of "fat" in his frame), and precision. His cinema was driven by the pursuit of an absolute leanness that would drive out any lingering connections to the sloppy, wheezing, fat figure of the cultural imaginary. Hitchcock certainly made films in order to domesticate and neutralize his childhood fears, but he also saw cinema as a proving ground, whereby he could show the many ways in which he was intellectually limber, stylistically economical, and refined. These compulsions to manifest a self divorced from the connotations of fatness helped produce the "genius" we enjoy in his cinema. We are incredibly fortunate to have at our disposal his entire body of work, in all of its tall, thin, and handsome dimensions. At least to this writer, he has proven his case.

1

Hitchcock's Hollywood diet

Alfred Joseph Hitchcock's 1939 relocation from his native London to Los Angeles set the stage for a surreal indoctrination into a culture he had only glimpsed through the refractions of the silver screen. Signing with SIP meant much more than leaving the homeland that had embraced him with growing enthusiasm as a national treasure over a fifteen-year directorial career. It meant more than adapting to new and cutting edge film technologies, more than submitting to the will of an erratic and headstrong studio boss. It also signaled his entrance into a milieu that demanded public, almost quotidian, access to his body. Consequently, it required a radical reassessment of his relationship to his body, and an intensification of self-surveillance and heightened self-consciousness.

In making the move to America, it is impossible to say how much Hitchcock had anticipated this rigorous negotiation of his celebrity persona. He discovered quickly that playing the Hollywood game required a new way of parsing the corporeal, and it made impossible the delusion—had he ever entertained one—of living or directing films with any sense of disembodiment. Between the mundane familiarity of *Jamaica Inn*—his last British production—and the jarring culture shock of *Rebecca*, where he began preproduction by sifting through hundreds of starlet screen tests, he had to acknowledge a new marketplace of glamorous signifying bodies, and in participating in the publicity for this DuMaurier adaptation, he would quickly learn that, for the first time in his forty years, *his* was also a body that mattered, both to the media and to the viewing public. Once solely the subject of his private frustration and anxiety, his corpulence was suddenly writ large, and it became startlingly connected to his public perception and, through his superiors' orchestrations, to his professional success.

The Americanization of Hitchcock's body was an ambivalent transformation, where the commodification of his fatness gave him purchase in the cult of charismatic celebrity, as a jovial avuncular, but it also magnified his feelings of shame and impotence, particularly when aggressive insults and more subtle insinuations about his body were used to manipulate him. The pages to come describe the pervasive and potent signifying powers of his body, used by *and* against him. Focusing on the first decade of Hitchcock's American life yields great insight into how his cultural legibility was rooted in his public, spectacular fatness.[1]

The second half of this chapter examines the relationship between Hitchcock and his first American employer David O. Selznick to suggest that throughout the 1940s, artistic control over Hitchcock's body of work was tautly, and in unsuspected ways, linked to control of his body's signification. Indeed, Hitchcock's body was implicated, and its meanings contested, at the center of many tumultuous business negotiations within SIP while he was under contract. This chapter will underwrite the endeavor of the following ones that explore Hitchcock's interior life, particularly as it both was influenced by, and made sense of, his fatness, and how that interior life found expression in his body of work.

The makings of a media giant

In his comprehensive biography, Patrick McGilligan rightly remarks that—unlike the American media—the British press was by and large respectful of Hitchcock in its reportage of his career, and usually refrained from any mention of his size or his weight, at least until he made his historic and ambivalently received move to America. In the 1920s and 1930s, Britain had not quite embraced motion pictures as part of its tabloid and celebrity gossip culture, preferring instead to focus on debutantes, royals, and stars of the theater. In stark contrast, America had by the late teens already cultivated a media industry—newspapers, magazines, fan clubs—devoted to film celebrity.

In his early days as title designer and even after easing into his first few directorial efforts for UFA in Berlin and Islington at home in London, Hitchcock likely gave little thought to receiving even a mention in the papers. It was the great success of his 1927 *The Lodger* that first put him on the radar of London publications, and by 1929's *Blackmail*, and *Murder!* the following year, his work was regularly followed by the *London Times, Bioscope*, and the *Daily Express*, among others. Most English coverage of the director was respectful, if not always celebratory, primarily addressing the production and release of his films; his frequent studio movement among Gainsborough, British International, and Gaumont British Picture Corporation also garnered attention.

The first notable departure from his usually harmonious relationship with the British media found its expression in a remark that Sidney Gilliat, cowriter with Frank Launder on 1938's *The Lady Vanishes*, made to the press after feeling slighted by the writing credit he was given. Hitchcock took umbrage at Gilliat's sour description of him as "a big bully who steals all the marbles."[2] Seeing this playground metaphor as a barely veiled reference to his weight, Hitchcock answered back in the press, and took time to get over the perceived insult. In retrospect, Hitchcock's offense at such an innocuous, off-the-cuff remark seems disproportionate, considering the slings and arrows of American publicity to come. If he had felt pricked by Gilliat, then his treatment in the United States must have been deeply penetrating, regardless of the thick (or, at least, calloused) skin he developed over the years.

Indeed, journalists in the United States seized on the spectacle of his size and peppered their introductory pieces with anecdotes of his remarkable appetite right away. In 1937, intrigued by American innovations in cinema, Hitchcock embarked on his first prospecting venture to the States in hopes of securing a picture deal with a Hollywood studio, or at least some promising contacts. After his first encounters with New York City's fourth estate, it became clear that reporters found their hook in his eating habits as well as his physique, and Hitchcock, to a large degree, was complicit in promoting this angle; at mealtime interviews, reporters attentively recorded his menu choices and appropriated the lighthearted quips he made about his girth for their often hyperbolic profiles of the director.

On this whirlwind New York visit he succeeded in making an indelible mark on the 21 Club, and unwittingly laid the foundation for America's tireless fascination with his appetite. In what may be described as the *primal scene* of his public identity as America's favorite fat man, Hitchcock dined with the *New York Herald Tribune*'s H. Allen Smith and, capitalizing on this perceived fascination with his gustatory potential, ordered his now legendary six-course meal: steak, followed by ice cream, repeated two more times, and washed down with brandies and three pots of English tea. The *Tribune* of course trumpeted this one-man orgy, delighting in the fact that after the meal, Hitchcock was taken to the cooler of the 21 Club to tour its meat offerings.

Smith's write-up of this 21 Club encounter included a moment of what biographer Donald Spoto has called Hitchcock's "uncharacteristic honesty." As an apparently impressed Smith turned the interview to the question of his appetites, Hitchcock thoughtfully confessed: "I find contentment from food. It's a mental process rather than a physical. There is as much anticipation in confronting good food as there is in going on a holiday, or seeing a good show. There are two kinds of eating—eating to sustain and eating for pleasure. I eat for pleasure."

In another interview a few days later, given to a Brooklyn reporter, he offhandedly observed, "I first started to put on weight when I took to drink."

His wife Alma Rèville, who dutifully monitored, and would at times restrict, his eating and drinking over the years, was notably absent from this exchange, and one wonders if Alma may have served a very useful purpose as buffer in much of his publicity.[3]

Hitchcock, of course, was savvy in realizing that this food-and-drink angle would make for good copy, but after returning to London, he was dismayed that in print, this interest in his Bacchanalian appetites eclipsed the celebration of his status as Britain's most promising director. Instead of being hailed as the next European to conquer Hollywood, he was cast as a "Falstaffian" who resembled "one of those jolly sultans in an *Esquire* cartoon," and perhaps most savagely, "a walking monument to the principle of uninhibited addiction to sack and capon, prime beef and flowing ale, and double helpings of ice cream."[4] Even more upsetting to him, no movie deal materialized to soften the blow. McGilligan identifies this visit as the exposure that produced the "first whiff of a Hitchcock caricature that would soon become the director's public face, for better or for worse." The "better" and the "worse" of this uneasy, but lasting marriage of director to fat caricature, is what this book aspires to narrate.

Hitch changed tactics in his visit a year later, careful not to curry favor with the press by playing up the indulgences of the previous visit. This time, in meeting the press at the 21 Club, he made sure to emphasize his sensible lunch of broiled lamb steak, cantaloupe, and pineapple, and to assure his companion of the press, "Mustn't get too heavy, you know? You've read those advertisements: 'When I meet a girl she always passes me by.'" (214). Hitchcock spoke of the ad as a sort of cautionary tale, but in truth it came closer to reflecting his own casual dynamic with women. Not only had he been "off the market" since his marriage to Alma in 1926, but his lifetime struggle with being overweight had generated a solid and rarely deviating self-perception of being far removed from the world of romance and desire.

Most of the major Hollywood studios—particularly MGM, Warner Brothers, and Paramount—had followed Hitchcock's English career throughout the 1930s with interest. With celebrity directors like Ernst Lubitsch and F. W. Murnau having emigrated to Hollywood in the 1920s, US film execs continued to surveil and mine the talents of European cinema, among them Fritz Lang in Germany, Rene Clair, Julien DuVivier, and Jean Renoir in France, and Hitch and compatriot Robert Stevenson in England. By 1932, a handful of Hitch's pictures—*Blackmail*, *Juno and the Paycock*, *Murder!*, and *The Skin Game*—had received American distribution, and that same year David O. Selznick received a cable from a representative in London raving that Hitchcock "[was] the best English director in England and made the finest English pictures made over there."[5] After the impressive box office successes of *The Man Who Knew Too*

Much (1934) and *The 39 Steps* (1935), Hitchcock looked like a sure thing for Hollywood recruitment. However, his follow-ups in the next two years (*The Secret Agent, Sabotage, Young and Innocent*) did not live up to the reputation he had begun to establish, and most American studios changed their minds about extending him an invitation.

With confidence somewhat restored by the feted release of *The Lady Vanishes*, Selznick, a former MGM exec now heading up his own SIP, stayed focused on what he sensed was a valuable acquisition. Before extending an offer, he confided in an associate, "There is very little doubt in my mind but that Hitchcock has already been sufficiently developed as a personality that we can get him for whatever top money is that the present market will afford."[6] Soon after, he secured a seven-year exclusive contract with Hitchcock. With the understanding that he would begin his Hollywood career helming either a *Titanic* epic or an adaptation of Daphne DuMaurier's *Rebecca*, Hitch relocated from London to Los Angeles with wife Alma, daughter Patricia, their cook, a secretary, and a couple of dogs in tow, and started on salary at Selznick International on April 10, 1939.

The arrival of the "300-Pound Prophet"

Almost immediately after Hitchcock's arrival in Los Angeles, the press came calling. Katharine Roberts, one of the first to capture Hitch in his new Hollywood habitat, published a lifestyle piece in *Collier's Weekly*, featuring the Hitchcock household, their daily routine, and their process of adapting to American life. Unsurprisingly, Hitchcock's weight and diet took center stage in her full-page article. She writes:

> [Hitchcock] thinks climbing stairs keeps his weight down. In the last half year he has lost thirty pounds, and he is anxious to report that he is not a heavy eater. In fact, he eats very little. Be that as it may. If you add his two hundred and sixty pounds to his wife's ninety five you haven't such a bad average.[7]

Framed with skepticism by Roberts, Hitch's claim to eat small to moderate portions would reappear in public media throughout his career. He intermittently publicized his weight loss efforts and often lamented that the self-discipline he exercised was never reflected in his physique.[8]

As late as 1956, Hitchcock exhibited a persistent desire to share with his reading public the frustrating disconnect between his diet and his appearance. In a relationship piece he wrote for *McCall's*, entitled "The Woman Who Knows

Too Much," he pays loving tribute to the many professional and domestic hats wife Alma wore throughout their marriage. He laments, "Contrary to what one would think from my measurements, I'm not a heavy eater. I'm simply one of those unfortunates who can accidentally swallow a cashew nut and put on thirty pounds right away."[9] Humor and hyperbole aside, Hitchcock's complaint addresses a real source of painful frustration that afflicted him throughout his life. Through the levity, we may hear the poignant protestation: *I don't deserve to be this fat.* In this optic, Roberts's dismissive "Be that as it may" is offered in the spirit of playful derision, yet it unknowingly engages a source of angst that was fundamental to Hitchcock's embodied identity.

I will later discuss Hitchcock's publicity and his general press promotion during the release of his first American film *Rebecca* as it was engineered by Selznick and SIP. His second release, *Foreign Correspondent*, filmed soon after in the middle of 1940, witnessed a sea change in the attitudes of the British press toward their truant Golden Boy. In America, *Foreign Correspondent*, just like his Oscar-winning *Rebecca*, garnered a lot of praise and was instantly popular; it too received a nomination for Best Picture in 1940. It was so successful, in fact, that Walter Wanger, the producer of *Correspondent* and the first studio head to receive Hitch by loan-out from SIP, entertained the idea of a sequel for several years after its release. He was hoping to bring Hitch back to work after completing his loan-out to RKO Pictures for *Suspicion* and *Mr. and Mrs. Smith*.

Overseas was a different story. *Correspondent* struck an especially dissonant chord with the British. England had declared war on Germany on September 3, 1939, and only five days after *Correspondent* finished shooting, the first Axis bombs fell on the United Kingdom, precipitating the Battle of Britain within a month.[10] The film's final scene depicts the blitz in London and a call to America to act as the last defense against fascism. "Hold on to your lights," Joel McCrea's protagonist broadcasts in the parting line of the film, "They're the only lights left in the world."

Hitchcock had been excused from British military service in the First World War, in 1917, with a C3 classification based on his obesity, which the examining doctor characterized as a glandular condition. In 1941, Hitch was eleven years over the draft age in England, but as a national figure, he was expected to show his patriotism, to return to his country and led by example. Obviously, his contract with Selznick made this gesture of loyalty impossible. Yet many were upset at their perceived abandonment by an ingrate who was now enjoying the luxuries of America rather than standing with his countrymen.

Michael Balcon of Gaumont Pictures, who took credit for building Hitch's career in England, shamed him in the press, referring to him not by name, but disparagingly as "a plump young junior technician," who was hiding out in

Hollywood from the dangers of war.[11] It is noteworthy that as ties of sympathy with his homeland frayed, so did the manners of British reportage, regarding his weight and size.[12] Interestingly, even a more sympathetic London newspaper could not refrain from mentioning his size: "It's obvious the celebrated and portly director would love to be over here [making films]—but alas! When you're tied to a producer, you're definitely not your own master!"

The animus against Hitchcock for abandoning Britain at its most vulnerable time, as well as the below-the-belt waistline humor, continued in England throughout the war, even after Hitchcock began his most dramatic weight loss regime. He was only partially redeemed by his voyage back to Europe to make two pro-Allied short propaganda films, *Bon Voyage* and *Aventure Malgache*, for France in 1944.

Although it is clear that Hitch was irritated, if not enraged, by the unflattering coverage of his weight, he rarely spoke publicly or at length about the reasons for his radical weight loss from 1942–45. His commitment to self-improvement appears to have been the convergence of several influences in both his personal and professional life. In a moment of reflective vulnerability and poignant disclosure, he spoke solemnly to the press of his jarring reaction to seeing a "grotesquely swollen man" in the reflection of a shop window, which he was loathe to recognize as his now 300-pound self. In his disgust and alarm at the "swollen man" presented before him, he committed himself to a strict daily regimen of coffee for breakfast and lunch, and steak and a small salad for dinner.

In December of 1943, even after he had been dieting with a great degree of commitment (and not a few lapses), Selznick received a telegram from the studio doctor, reporting that Hitchcock had been denied insurance coverage by their reissuance companies, and by the Occidental Insurance Co., finding that "1. Although Mr. Hitchcock has lost considerable weight, he is still overweight. 2. Mr. Hitchcock has a very bad hernia. 3. Investigation reveals that his heart is enlarged 16%." These companies, however, said that, if he successfully underwent an operation for his hernia (which, of course, he did—sixteen years later, in 1957), then they would consider reissuing insurance coverage to him.

A year before this worrying check-up, Hitchcock lost both his mother Emma (1942) and brother William, who remained back in London, to illness and suicide, respectively. The death of William, who was nine years Alfred's senior, very likely occasioned a sober reassessment of his habits of consumption. His next New Year's resolution was a vow to lose 100 pounds. Donald Spoto, in his *The Dark Side of Genius*, ruminates at length about the impact of these two deaths on his conscience, his feelings of guilt at having left his extended family behind in a time of war and in his mother's declining health. As Spoto would have it, these unresolved guilty feelings surrounding their estrangement and his powerlessness to help or be near her in her final days would fester and grow, shaping the hostile and bizarre representations of mothers and maternity that characterize his late films (*Psycho, The Birds, Marnie*) and even those made earlier, such as *Notorious* and *Strangers On a Train*.

It is noteworthy that Hitchcock was angered by his authorized biographer's reportage of the circumstances leading up to his brother's death. Hitchcock, in fact, asked John Russell Taylor to remove from his manuscript the claim that William's death had been hastened by drinking. "Do you really need that?" he beseechingly asked Taylor, recognizing that it not only besmirched his brother's memory, but also colored his own reputation, already saturated with stories about his own heavy drinking and eating. McGilligan and Spoto report that Hitchcock's alcohol consumption often skyrocketed in times of stress and uncertainty, and there seem to be ample anecdotes to confirm this correlation. And of course the press was as ever on hand to remark on these indulgences.

As Hitchcock was shooting *Foreign Correspondent*, his second American film, he was struggling with finances, unhappy with the contractual allowance provided by Selznick, and overwhelmed with financing a new Hollywood lifestyle. Samson Raphaelson, who cowrote 1941's *Suspicion* (with Joan Harrison and Reville), later reminisced that he and Hitch had been drunk during most of their planning of the film, with Hitch, never without a hand extended, offering a pitcher of gin and orange juice. While this flippant characterization is no doubt an exaggeration, *Correspondent* star Joel McCrea reported at the same time to the press that Hitchcock would polish off a pint of champagne at lunch and then nap throughout the afternoon shoot. His oft-repeated account of Hitch waking up at the end of a scene, inquiring as to whether it was printable (to which McCrea replied in the affirmative), gave further credence to reports that he habitually fell asleep in public.

However much it made headlines, this kind of consumption in no way characterized his behavior throughout all film shoots. Just two years later, those on *Saboteur* would depict him as always lucid and focused, and small in appetite. Peter Viertel, who cowrote *Saboteur* with Joan Harrison and Dorothy Parker, fondly recalls Hitch's hobby of collecting menus from exquisite restaurants, which he would recite to family and dining companions: "The menu was full of succulent delights, and Hitch would get his kicks just out of reading it, but then lunch would be Spartan, maybe a salad with a side of lamb. . . . You never saw him drunk." In fact, McGilligan reports that others close to him at this time remarked upon the disconnect between his weight and his food intake, leading them to believe that perhaps his wartime diagnosis of a glandular condition may have been accurate.

In reading the compendium of available Hitchcock anecdotes, it is remarkable how many actors, writers, technicians, and friends recall memories of Hitchcock that revolve around food or their perception of his size at the time. Hume Cronyn, a collaborator of Hitchcock's for over ten years who acted in *Shadow of a Doubt*, *Lifeboat*, and two episodes of *Hitchcock Presents*, and cowrote *Rope* and *Under Capricorn*, shared his first and most lasting impression of Hitch with Patrick McGilligan: "He wore a double-breasted suit; four fingers of each hand were buried in his armpits, but his thumb stuck straight up. He weighed close to 300 pounds and looked remarkably like a genial Buddha."

Recalling the elaborate meals that Hitchcock planned for family, cast, and visiting friends at the Occidental Hotel in Santa Rosa throughout their location shoot of *Shadow*, Cronyn recalls, "Martinis preceded a menu he specifically ordered; the lamb, he directed, had to be pink." While his reminiscence of principal photography on *Shadow* comes across as a fond and affectionate recollection—and repeatedly Hitchcock himself would nostalgically recall the smooth and convivial vibe of this shoot—Cronyn caps off the memory with the ambivalent observation, "The martinis, the meal, his immense weight, to say nothing of the day's work, would take their toll until Hitch's chins would rest on his chest, and he would start to snore gently."[13] He reports that Alma, ever the vigilant companion, would chuck him on the nose to wake him at such moments.

Hitchcock referred back proudly and often to his 1943 film *Shadow of a Doubt*, and both American audiences and critics hailed it as a very strong thriller. The British press, however, embittered by his absence and still agitated perhaps by the perceived insult of *Foreign Correspondent*, toed the line that he had sold out, was subordinating strong technique to romance and superficial Hollywood glitz. C. A. LeJeune of the *London Observer* used the headline "Stout Fellow" for her review of *Shadow*, and in it, likened him to Orson Welles, their commonality based not on their prodigious talent, but on their fluctuating waistline. The review quipped, "Statisticians who are interested in the relations between avoirdupois and the study of crime may care to observe that the falling curve of [Hitchcock's] waistcoat has been followed by a corresponding fall in the curve of his films." Even as Hitchcock lost a substantial amount of weight, his size was still used to denigrate his work and to decry his choice to relocate to Hollywood.

Selznick's fat commodity

In what follows, I take a closer look at the nine-year working relationship between Alfred Hitchcock, David O. Selznick, and the executives at Selznick

International. The contentious relationship between Hitchcock and Selznick has been well-documented, receiving great attention in the work of McGilligan, Taylor, and Spoto, and most prominently in the monograph devoted to it: *Hitchcock and Selznick* by Leonard Leff. From artistic differences about the process of adaptation surrounding *Rebecca*, to the length of time Hitchcock spent shooting, to casting choices, to film assignments, to salary, the relationship rarely saw a true détente.

Rather than recapitulating the struggles for power that punctuated their collaboration here, I intend to focus on the ways that Hitchcock's weight, size, and appetites became tropes that fueled Hitchcock publicity, saturated their interpersonal exchanges, and mobilized their conflicting creative agendas in conscious and unconscious ways. In this admittedly unique assessment of the professional and personal dynamic at SIP, I resist consigning Selznick to Gilliat's earlier "big bully who steals all the marbles," nor do I limit Hitchcock to the role of perennially taunted fat kid. I do, however, maintain that Selznick and his cronies used Hitch's vulnerability in strategic ways: first, as a means of building a flamboyant public persona in which spectators and readers could find memorable amusement; and secondly, invoking his weight and size to make him comply with their wishes and to shame and disarm him when contract disputes arose. Hitchcock's fatness, and the uses others made of it, actually shaped the course of his cinematic career to a fascinating extent.

Hitchcock was contractually bound to SIP from his arrival to Los Angeles in 1939, until 1947, when he completed work on *The Paradine Case*. At this point, he began producing his own films with Sidney Bernstein under the auspices of Transatlantic Pictures, which they had formed discreetly—though not discreetly enough to avoid the unhappy detection of Selznick—in 1945, in anticipation of his freedom from SIP.[14] During the course of his contractual obligation, Hitchcock made three films directly for Selznick—*Rebecca*, *Spellbound*, and *Paradine*—and was loaned out to neighboring studios for seven: Walter Wanger for *Foreign Correspondent*, RKO for *Suspicion*, *Mr. and Mrs. Smith*, and *Notorious*, Universal for *Saboteur* and *Shadow of a Doubt*, and Twentieth Century Fox for *Lifeboat*.

Selznick was undoubtedly wise to bring Hitchcock on board SIP. Though he time and again expressed dismay with the output of their collaboration—most pointedly, at the speed with which Hitch could complete a picture—he profited greatly from their collaboration. By 1943, Hitch was loaned out to Twentieth Century Fox for a forty-week stint at 7,500 dollars a week, and a prorated 3,750 dollars for each additional week. Whereas Hitchcock started with RKO in 1941 at 3,000 dollars a week, by their final collaboration in 1946, he was netting Selznick double that, at a weekly 6,000 dollars.

It is undeniable that, from the very start of their partnership, beginning with their tumultuous production of *Rebecca*, Selznick capitalized on the American media's fascination with Hitchcock's weight that had been established in his early trips to America, several years before he was recruited to the States. Recognizing that his size could be used as an idiosyncratic hook to market him memorably to the American public, he ensured that Hitch's studio publicity was playfully punctuated with an affectionate sense of humor regarding his rotundity. It is with Selznick's blessing that headlines such as Alva Johnston's well-known "300-Pound Prophet Comes to Hollywood" proliferated.[15]

Selznick's compliance with and catering to the American public's persistent fixation on Hitchcock's weight is evident in the publicity photographs for which Hitchcock posed to promote *Rebecca*. Four publicity stills and their captions illustrate perfectly how Selznick International used the spectacle of his weight to promote his public image. Photographer Don Roberts refers to Hitchcock as a "239-pound Englishman" in one caption, a "239-pound director" in two others, and in the fourth, remarks, "'Hitch,' who likes to talk about movies and himself, doesn't mind allusions to his 239 pounds." One picture is entitled "Heavyweight in Light Mood." In it, Hitchcock poses with an inflatable plastic barbell while suppressing a yawn, suggesting the ease with which he (pretends to) carry the weight. The prop is straight from the film, where the also-portly actor Nigel Bruce carries it as part of a Samson getup he wears to a costume ball. In both situations, the humor derives from the spectacle of a flabby man trying—and failing—to perform the illusion of great strength and easy masculinity.

In the second photo, Roberts seems to be reaching for an allusion to Hitchcock's weight, but manages with the feeble caption, "Props Can Take It." Posed simply sitting down in a re-creation of the film's dining room, Hitchcock "tests a chair on the set of *Rebecca*," the obvious implication being that he is likely to break furniture by applying his weight to it. A third photo shows Hitchcock taking a tea break, mentioning the 239-pound Englishman's preference to make his own tea while directing (which was not true). A fourth still bears the caption, "Master of Menace," with the labored description of Hitch as, "Unmenacing himself except when it comes to eating." Thus the banal and uninspired one-dimensionality of his public portrayal—a portrayal generated by his own production company—demonstrates the casual, quotidian nature of the publicity that associated Hitchcock with spectacular fatness. What had caught on at the 21 Club several years prior had now been codified in the public imaginary through Selznick's machinations.

In many regards, through their 1938 contract, Hitchcock became the property—not simply the *intellectual* or *creative* property—of Selznick International. A 1942 press release minces no words in recognizing the proprietary relationship: "David still owns the rotund master of chills and suspense, and rents him out to other studios at a profit."[16] Selznick not only controlled Hitchcock's working conditions, the terms of his many loan-outs to other studios, and the kinds of pictures he was making; he also controlled the rights to his likeness and his name. A memo from the legal department of Paramount Pictures, dated May 6, 1941, underscores the tightness of SIP's grip on their *wunderkind* director. In this missive, Paramount sought permission to use Hitchcock's name in the dialogue of Preston Sturges's comedy *Sullivan's Travels.*

The memo, addressed to SIP Executive Vice-President Daniel T. O'Shea, reads as follows:

> We are enclosing the page from Preston Sturges's script which contains the scene in which Mr. Hitchcock's name is used. In this new shooting script, you will note there is a slight change. The girl now asks: Is Hitchcock as fat as they say he is? And the director replies: Fatter. We would appreciate an early reply, inasmuch as this picture is about to go into production.[17]

This memo followed on the heels of one sent three days prior, also addressed to Dan O'Shea, which was more succinct. "Will you please confirm on the attached copy that you have no objection to our proposed use of Hitchcock's name and also secure his personal consent at the place indicated, and return the same to me? Very truly yours." While the personal consent of Hitchcock seems to have been a prerequisite, the decision was clearly a corporate one, predicated on SIP's assumption of control over his image and name. Operating on the principle that all publicity is good publicity, SIP okayed the reference, and the dialogue stayed in the picture.

In all instances of SIP's loan-outs of Hitchcock, the contracts governing his temporary work at each studio contained precise stipulations restricting the "borrowing" producer's ability to use his name and likeness. While this sort of clause was normal procedure for the loan-outs of actors, and perhaps the occasional procedure for directors, the tight restrictions of SIP's contracts are especially resonant, given Selznick's great care in regulating Hitch's public exposure.

In SIP's May 1, 1944, contract with Vanguard Films, the coproducer of *Spellbound* with Selznick's *own* company, the agreement stipulates,

> You agree that you will not advertise or announce, or permit the advertisement or announcement of the name, or use, or permit the use of, the likeness of the Director in the general advertising or paid publicity issued by you to announce the names of directors rendering services

> for you, or in connection with any commercial or advertising tie-ups, but that any announcements of the Director's name shall be made only in connection with and relating to said photoplays.

The contract seems intended to prevent Hitchcock's perceived identification or affiliation with any studio except Selznick's. Hence, it was important to him that Hitchcock be seen as part of the SIP stable, and that the public be reminded perpetually of Selznick's coup in bringing the director to Hollywood.

The executives at SIP concerned themselves also with the kind of company Hitchcock was keeping in the public eye. Hitch was very interested in bringing Joseph Cotten on board for *Shadow of a Doubt*, and of course he eventually got his way. However, when O'Shea heard of this, he held a meeting in Selznick's absence, worrying over who had loaned him out to Hitchcock, and whether Selznick had signed him personally. He expressed trepidation about how it would look for the press to publicize Hitch's association with Cotten, whose name at the time was taboo in the Hearst papers because of his role in *Citizen Kane*.

Selznick and his colleagues' strong desire to control Hitchcock's career choices, as well as his affiliations, manifests itself in the many memos that circulated among them. One case in point is the vigilance with which they watched Hitchcock's moves after he had approached London SIP exec Sig Marcus about the possibility of employing his brother William as a sort of surrogate through which he could pick up additional income. Marcus had given him a resolute "No," and had immediately informed the US execs of what they considered an egregious act of ingratitude, disloyalty, and greed.

Their concern for his scheme shines through in a rather cryptic telegram that Myron Selznick's London agent Harry Ham sent to Marcus, reading: "Had dinner with ALFRED HITCHCOCK last night and, strange as it may be to you and me, he appeared to be under control."[18] The idea of having Hitchcock "under control" crops up in many SIP communications. In a telegram sent a few years later, in April of 1945, from Selznick to O'Shea, Selznick writes:

> It is important that we have no obligation to Mr. Hitchcock beyond payment of money. . . . We should be perfectly free, if occasion rose, not to use him, or to substitute a story after he had worked on one, or to substitute another director, or anything else. Otherwise, we are at his mercy.

Control over artistic decisions and financial transactions was clearly a sine qua non for Selznick, and when this feeling of control was challenged, he tightened the reins.

Part of Selznick's method of reining Hitchcock in became apparent when, after the impressive performance of *Rebecca* and *Foreign Correspondent*, Hitch was offered a chance to direct the first episode of the new radio program *Suspense*, a series that would thrive on CBS radio for the next twenty years. Hitchcock and Selznick agreed that Hitch could both host and direct the first installment of the show, provided the program would publicize the opening of *Foreign Correspondent* the following month.

They chose an adaptation of Hitch's first great success in Britain, *The Lodger*, and the episode was a hit. Based on its ratings and the amount of fan mail received, CBS extended an offer to Hitchcock to come on board as full-time host of the show. This transition from director to host was not unprecedented; esteemed director Cecil B. DeMille had been hosting and promoting the Lux Radio Theater since 1936, and the deal was quite lucrative. As host, he would have assumed the role of "Master of Suspense."[19] (Obviously, this moniker was not wasted.) This offer was rejected by execs of SIP outright. Hitch had not even pushed for the position, understanding very well the strictures of his corporate obligations. In a telling memo to Selznick on August 17, 1940, O'Shea affirms his aversion to Hitchcock's taking up CBS' offer.

> On the subject of Hitch's going on the radio . . . I would have turned him down cold even though the considerations which you mention, such as building up Hitch's name and his gross and publicity for us, are considerations with merit and not to be cast aside lightly. I feel, however, that we would be creating a Frankenstein monster. *In size Hitch is a monster now, but imagine him as a Frankenstein monster*![20]

This communication between O'Shea and Selznick reveals an insecurity they shared regarding Hitchcock's becoming a Hollywood entity that could no longer be kept in line by SIP, and also suggests a fear that the great demand for his services could make him arrogant, ambitious, and harder to keep in compliance with SIP's professional plans for him.

The memo also indicates their preoccupation with Hitch's weight. Fat jokes about Hitchcock between Selznick and his colleagues were a staple of interoffice communications, and more muted insinuations of his size appeared in direct correspondences with Hitch, usually in an attempt to humble or demean him, or to deflate his sense of entitlement in asking for more money or latitude in his filming schedule. The juvenile banter here, which describes Hitchcock's size as "monstrous," amounts to the posturing of a bully—a tactic that Selznick and O'Shea would adopt frequently—and appears to have deflected a genuine fear that he was getting "too big for his britches."

The knowledge that Hitchcock's Achilles' heel was almost any pointed reference to his size, whether in the form of a joke or in the guise of concern for his health, produced a juvenile arsenal for SIP to wield at will, especially in times of tension and conflict. A striking instance of this aggressive shaming occurred early in their working relationship. In May of 1940, just a year after emigrating, Hitchcock found himself in dire financial straits. Between setting down roots in Los Angeles with his family and dealing with unfinished financial business back in England, which included a production company that needed to be liquidated, he began to panic over his inability simply to make ends meet.

Contributing to this dilemma was his difficulty securing funds from his accounts in England due to war restrictions. To soften the financial blow of his transition, he hoped that Selznick would agree to let him augment his income by directing an additional picture outside his contract. In a radio interview around this time, Hitchcock imprudently and extemporaneously discoursed at length about the great expense involved in his relocation, and intimated that SIP was not providing him with sufficient compensation to make the transition an easy one. After receiving word that Hitch had in essence publicly complained about his treatment from David and brother Myron (his agent), a mortified O'Shea, acting on Selznick's behalf, sent a memo chastising the director for his indiscretion and ingratitude. He snarkily concluded the memo, with a disingenuous inquiry of concern: "*How's the metabolism?*" This kind of remark—a cheap shot wrapped in a thin veneer of politesse—came to characterize the veiled antagonism so often expressed by his first Hollywood employers.

Occasionally Hitchcock himself would invoke his size in his interactions with Selznick and O'Shea, usually to diffuse a tense situation with comedy or to self-deprecate as a demonstration of his powerlessness while under contract. Unfortunately, his willingness to participate in the ongoing fat joke only seemed to point to its effectiveness as a strategy to curb any of Hitch's desires that ran counter to the plans and the vision of Selznick.

In the May of 1940, the same month that O'Shea made his dig at his metabolism, Hitchcock sent a Western Union telegram to Selznick. In it, he beseeches only half-jokingly, "Please David if you have a shred of love for me at all answer this plaintive cry of your devoted servant who has lost a lot of weight through anxiety and diet. HITCH."[21] In his despair, Hitch tempers what seems to be an authentic supplication with a bit of the court jester routine, thereby playing into the caricature that Selznick and compadres had already fashioned and exploited. Putting himself in the role of damsel in distress, who "has lost a lot of weight," he facetiously courts the ridiculous proposition that weight loss would be unhealthy for him.

Three days later, O'Shea responded to Hitchcock's entreaty, indicating that a loan could be arranged. He reminds Hitch—as he had often in the past—that Selznick had stood by him when other studios had lost interest in recruiting him to America. He callously mentions the derision that his final British film *Jamaica Inn* met with in Hollywood, and again suggests that gratitude for SIP's meticulous care is what he owes them. He of course picks up on Hitchcock's fat joke, answering back in kind: "Advise me whether you need any temporary help until my return and accept my sympathies over your loss of weight which however I am confident you will rebuild on adulation which I am sure you will continue to receive and which we both know you so *largely* deserve." O'Shea plays along with Hitchcock's assumption of the role of a wilting flower, facetiously depicting his weight loss as an undesirable outcome and curiously, he seems to correlate Hitch's regaining weight with receiving professional kudos for his filmmaking. The insinuation here is that Hitchcock becomes fatter the more the viewing public "spoils" him with praise. This continuation of the memo's original joke is just one of several instances in which Selznick and O'Shea conflate Hitchcock's fatness with his inflated sense of self-worth as an artist.

A year earlier, for example, Selznick had felt threatened by other studios' interest in him and in a memo to O'Shea, he expressed his concerns. "I hope that Hitch isn't getting additionally *fat-headed* as a result." It is clear that Selznick means he worries that Hitch will grow "big-headed," in the sense of becoming conceited, rather than "fat-headed," or fatuous. It is noteworthy that his inclination is to use the word "fat." This seemingly reflexive, probably unconscious, resorting to the language of fatness crops up in Selznick's correspondences often.

In 1945, when Selznick felt that Hitch was racking up runaway production costs for *Notorious,* he angrily wrote to another associate: "Hitchcock has the indian sign on us and on Dan [O'Shea] particularly. Just because Hitchcock uses up a big *fat* chair in Dan's office and distracts him from other work is no excuse for paying him almost a thousand dollars per day." A year later, when O'Shea neglected to take him off the payroll when he took a trip to New York City, Selznick admonished him. "He certainly has an Indian sign on you—a great big *fat* one!" In addition to referring to Hitchcock's manipulative nature (the repeated "indian sign"), the repetition of "fat" in these different contexts indicates that his temper habitually led him back to a disgust with Hitchcock's fatness, evincing a sense of Selznick's internalized fat-phobia.

Other correspondences between Selznick and O'Shea indicate clearly their perception of Hitchcock as, at different times, slow and greedy, and their descriptions of them in these regards, alternately bemused and accusatory, become connotatively linked with their ideas about his appetite and his size.[22] After Hitchcock took an afternoon off from shooting, supposedly because he was angry at not having cornered a larger percentage of his loan-out to RKO, O'Shea penned an impressively long and scathing disciplinary letter to Hitch which he never sent. In it, he makes clear his displeasure.

> You have neither the legal nor moral right to knock off for an afternoon for which you were receiving a very *heavy* payment. . . . Hitch, I think it is time that you took stock, and realized how increasingly difficult it is becoming for us to meet your growing reputation for slowness and for extravagance. . . . I can't think that it would be very good business on my part to cut you in on profits and then stand all the losses, even though we have done this with the bonuses we have already given you, as a gesture which apparently procured no gratitude, but only *further appetite*.

O'Shea goes on to compare Hitchcock's circumstances with other European directors—Clair, Lang, DuVivier, and Renoir—whose careers, upon coming to work in Hollywood, had not been nearly as lucrative as Hitchcock's had been, under the careful and generous guidance of Selznick International. "Whereas Clair was in five times the demand that you were before either of you came over, today he is having difficulty getting any kind of work," O'Shea writes, adding, "And Renoir, the master director of *The Grande Illusion* [*sic*], is utterly miserable, and from all reports faces a repetition of the Clair incident."[23]

O'Shea's passionate, somewhat manic letter illuminates a chain of connotations that link together the rhetorics of excess of both his and Selznick's communications. Hitchcock's fatness is linked variously with his slowness, his extravagance (not knowing when to stop), his greed (tellingly figured as his "appetite"), his intractability, his ingratitude (the infantilizing image of the ungrateful brat rears its head often), and his lack of self-discipline. In grounding all of his perceived deficiencies in the language of his fatness and by loading most of their communications with words such as *fat*, *large*, *heavy*, *excessive*, and *slow*, Selznick and O'Shea played upon Hitchcock's deepest insecurities, deploying shame to curb his aspirations outside of SIP and to suggest that he was getting more than he deserved. After O'Shea expressed regret in not sending the missive to Hitchcock, Selznick advised him to send it if he wanted to, reasoning that the truth would be "out there," as opposed to gossip, "since we all know what a *big mouth* Hitch has." Another dig at Hitchcock's lack of restraint punctuates his advice.

It may seem like selective over-reading or willful projection to identify any one of these various uses of *fat*, *large*, *heavy*, *slow*, *big-mouthed*, and other such words in SIP communications as evidence of conscious or unconscious fat-phobia, or of a semantic conspiracy to wrest the psychological upper hand from the "Master of Suspense" through shame or abjection. Yet, in my researching of the Selznick archive, and in my assessment of it here, I find the cumulative effect of these utterances compelling, and the many repetitions of words that connote fat, excess, and greed, simply cannot be ignored.

Hitchcock's previously elaborated decision to undergo a life-altering diet in 1943, following the death of his mother and brother, prompted also by his doctor's earnest warnings about his health risks, met with an interesting response on Selznick's part. While he often joked about Hitchcock's size and evoked his weight in a shaming capacity, he rarely echoed the health concerns of SIP's studio physician.[24] However, he *did* express concern when Hitchcock began to carry out his radical weight loss plan successfully. In an interoffice memo to O'Shea in May of 1943, he writes:

> I am sincerely and seriously worried about Hitch's fabulous loss of weight. I do hope he has a physician as otherwise we are liable to get a shock one morning about a heart attack or something of the sort. I think you ought to have a frank talk about this with Hitch.

This memo, where Selznick seems to be evincing concern for the weight loss of his associate, is bizarre for several reasons. First, Selznick's "hope [that] he has a physician" comes across as disingenuously flippant. Certainly he was aware that Hitchcock was being closely monitored by the studio's physician. The previously mentioned issues with Hitch's insurance coverage would necessitate this. In fact, from 1942 onward, Hitch met weekly with a physician to have his vital signs checked.

Secondly, there is an interesting ambivalence expressed, in that Hitchcock's weight loss is both "fabulous" and a potential cause for concern. Certainly, rapid weight loss poses some degree of cardiac risk, and it is not necessarily unusual to express concern for the drastic nature of his diet. Yet the equally concerning 300 pounds that Hitch had accumulated on his 5′ 6″ frame curiously never became part of Selznick's agenda. The accounts of Leff, Spoto, and McGilligan and the explicitness, scope, and detail of Selznick's own thousands of existent memos make it clear that Selznick was a conscientious and energetic micromanager. Perhaps most illustrative of this management style is the fact that the thinness of Ingrid Bergman's eyebrows was an action item at an August 1942 board meeting. One has to wonder why he did not express concern for the undeniable cardiac risk that his number one recruit's morbid obesity posed.

This concern that Selznick felt for Hitchcock's weight loss continued at least until 1945. In a May 23 memo to his in-house legal counsel Richard Hungate, Selznick is very vague about the nature of his most recent point of negotiation with Hitchcock, but he mentions O'Shea and Hitchcock in the following: "If Dan thinks we can accomplish a better result by my telephoning Hitchcock, I will do so; but tell him for the love of pete to 'DRINK A MALTED.'" Two years after his first expression of worry over Hitchcock's weight loss, he was clearly still preoccupied with the matter. In fact, by this time, he had gone from expressing concern to instructing Hitch (even if jokingly) to take steps to maintain his weight, certainly not to lose any more.

One possible explanation for both Selznick's inattention to the periods of Hitchcock's substantial weight gain and for the puzzling intervention that occurred when he was, in fact, *losing* weight, is that weight loss for Hitchcock meant diverging from the image of the plump, avuncular auteur that Selznick had worked so hard to commodify. A suddenly svelte Hitchcock was a (literally) unknown quantity on the Hollywood market. The radical change in his appearance may have caused a collective cognitive dissonance, and perhaps the charismatic persona that America had come to embrace would have disappeared and, with it, his fans' enthusiasm for their "300-pound prophet," for their "stout fellow."

A darker hypothesis would be that the executives at SIP intuited, consciously or not, that retaining control over Hitchcock's productivity and loyalty was more easily accomplished when his weight made him vulnerable and thereby chastened and compliant. The notion that a rise in his self-esteem might promote a boost in his self-assertion and resolve could only have caused them consternation. Hitchcock was locked into a contract with Selznick for those seven years, but contracts are not unbreakable, as concerned buddy Carole Lombard pointed out to him when she sensed his anxiety and unhappiness on the set of *Mr. and Mrs. Smith* (1941). Perhaps, success in his diet might make him feel more capable of change on a larger scale, more entitled, and less susceptible to the enfeebling playground taunts to which he was often subjected in his Selznick years.

Without a doubt, Hitchcock realized that becoming an American icon entailed much more than producing quality films. He understood, by the time he arrived in America, or shortly thereafter, that his reputation and chances for upward mobility on the Hollywood ladder were based on his assuming the role of the endearing, accessible, odd uncle. This iconic fashioning that Selznick set in motion, and with which Hitchcock dutifully complied, I argue, was instrumental in molding his career, and not just the business side of it. In the chapters that follow, I revisit his films with an eye toward his cinematic preoccupations with food and drink, with consumption and elimination, with bodies, size, proportion, and their ties to sex and romance, love and acceptance. I hope to demonstrate that Hitchcock's fatness and how it played out in his life did not stunt him as an artist and a person, nor did it constrain his creativity, but instead both reflected and set in motion a fascinating assortment of fantasies, nightmares, and riddles, many of which found their voice and bodies in his great cinemascape.

I also stand by my earlier *caveat* not to limit Selznick's role in the saga to the bully on the playground, behind whom the lesser antagonists posture and taunt. While aspects of their long collaboration were a source of disappointment for both of them, the fact remains that they accomplished a great deal, creating impressive and lasting cinematic monuments. What is more, the fact remains that Selznick did promote and nurture Hitchcock's career. He put forward the 10,000 dollars needed to liquidate Hitchcock Baker Productions Ltd., Hitchcock's English production company of ten years. He also arranged thoughtful gifts—for instance, he sent Hitchcock on a Palm Beach vacation in the latter's first year of employment. It is somewhat moving to note that one of his business items on a 1940 board meeting agenda read: "Alfred Hitchcock: Development of Hitchcock with the hope that he will become the most important directing figure in the business." Through the years of crossed wires and clenched fists, Selznick in no small way contributed to this becoming an eventual reality.

For those sympathetic to Hitchcock's plight in his early Hollywood years, there is, perhaps, a gratifying coda to the episodes narrated above, a symbolic answering back to Selznick and company's degradation of him, to the frequent manipulation of his bodily fears and the evocation of shame toward which he naturally gravitated. In 1956, Hitchcock's career and his public reception were thriving, on the heels of his healthily successful *Rear Window*, *Dial M for Murder*, *To Catch a Thief*, and *The Man Who Knew Too Much*. *Alfred Hitchcock Presents* had launched to a receptive television audience, and the energetic preparation for *Vertigo* had begun. Hitchcock was now being happily represented by MCA and alternating productions at Warner Brothers/First National and Paramount, when his old boss Selznick came a-calling.

Selznick still owned four of Hitch's films from the 1940s, and in an effort to drum up publicity for their rerelease, asked permission to use his famous eight-stroke profile caricature, now seen weekly by television audiences. Through agent Herman Citron, one of his reps at MCA, Hitchcock gave his answer: a resounding "No." The gesture was just one of the antagonistic slights that he and Selznick traded after the dissolution of their highly charged partnership, but there is something satisfying about his solid insistence that he finally be in control of the circulation of his body's image, and under what auspices.[25]

Hitchcock's refusal to accommodate a man who, just over a decade earlier, had exercised his legal authority to okay a fat joke at his expense—a joke released for the consumption of countless thousands of spectators globally—seems to be an empowering act of self-assertion rather than silly contrariness. Hitchcock may never have arrived at a place of comfort and peace with his size, whether in his private life or in his public presentation. Yet, the prerogative of choosing more often when and how to frame his body in various contexts must have been sweet relief and a slice of welcome liberation in his post-Selznick years.

2

The Hitchcock cameo: Fat self-fashioning and cinematic belonging

At the height of his popularity, Hitchcock was perhaps as renowned for the cameo appearances he made in his films as he was for the films themselves. While the cameos went largely unremarked by American audiences in the 1940s, by the early to mid-1950s, spectators had learned to look for the director's brief appearances.[1] At this point, the game of searching for the director became *de rigueur* for moviegoers, so much so that Hitchcock worried that the preoccupation with "finding Hitchcock" was detracting from his audience's narrative engagement, and consequently made sure to place these cameos early in the film. David Sterritt, in his *The Films of Alfred Hitchcock*, is one of the first Hitchcock critics to appreciate the complexity of the textual play that Hitchcock's cameos occasion, both as visual markers of the director's relation to his own characters and to the diegesis of his making, and as symptom of his personal need to engage with his textual world and have that engagement witnessed by his audiences.[2] Sterritt glosses the contributions of two scholars who have likewise taken seriously the semiotics of the cameo: Tom Ryall's observation that the cameo constitutes "that most familiar mark of Hitchcock's personalization of his films," generating savvy "qualities of self-consciousness" that depart from the purported "anonymity" associated with classical cinema; and Ronald Christ's characterization of the cameos as instances of *parabasis*, moments of "illusion-breaking" dramatic rupture, as in Greek comedy's choral direct address to the spectator.[3]

In his incisive account of the Hitchcock cameos, Sterritt makes the case for their significance beyond personalizing signature and parabasic disruption, reasoning that in addition to providing "self-publicizing jokes and ironic punctuations," and apart from their "illusion-breaking qualities," the cameos also disclose "Hitchcock's deep-seated wish not only to speak *through*, but to become physically integrated *with*, his films." He persuasively elaborates on the nature of these directorial wishes, first asserting Hitchcock's desire to not only "wink and wave at the audience," but to sardonically "comment on the action in some small, sly way"; second, noting Hitchcock's "wish to approach and 'keep an eye on' his characters"; and third, describing a "signal to his audience (which normally receives the message on a subliminal level) that he is the presiding spirit of his films."[4] Sterritt adds that the cameo, together with the presence of cinematic "surrogates" for Hitchcock—sometimes characters, sometimes object which bespeak a Hitchcockian point of view in his physical absence—evince his desire for a kind of fusion with the film's world.

In addition to Sterritt's astute assessments of the functions, both psychic and narrative, of the Hitchcock cameo, I would like to suggest in this chapter that his cameos generate what I will call a *mesogetic space*, meaning that his appearances are "intrusions" that do not rupture the diegesis entirely, nor do they stand squarely outside it in discrete isolation.[5] Rather, the cameos occupy a narrative middle ground that generates both irony and intimacy. That is, the cameo performs in both directions, within and outside of the narrative's space, permitting the kind of intertextual readings that enhance Hitchcock's filmic role through a consideration of how he signifies as celebrity in the world of the spectator.[6] Hitchcock's presence in the mesogesis inflects the film text, as Sterritt allows, in order to provide nuance to, or commentary on, the world of the film. It also projects outward, to convey to the audience a momentary ironic confluence of filmic and extra-filmic realities, and the sense of Hitchcock's solidarity with, and more importantly, *belonging to* the cast *and* the characters of his production. The cameo's gestures "outward" toward the audience were important to Hitchcock, I argue, in their imparting a sense of tradition and continuity across the course of his cinematic career. As his many anecdotes about the origin of his cameos demonstrate, his continuation of the cameo appearance throughout his career pays reverent homage to his early days of small English ensemble productions, in which he felt a fraternal part of a creative collectivity. This is a feeling he did not always experience in some of his larger, more sweeping American productions, where the crew was exponentially bigger and dispersed. The cameo then nostalgically brought him back in touch with these early experiences of ensemble and fraternal teamwork.

By extension, the cameo as a tradition in his filmmaking marked his place in a collectivity which became more difficult to conceptualize in his later, high-budget, widely diffuse American productions, which sprawled due to evolving technologies, the scope of his projects, and the exponential growth of production crew. In addition to their bridging the modesty of his early productions with the grandiosity of his later ones, these cameos were important to Hitchcock, in that his appearances constituted proof of the *cinematicity* of his body. Sterritt writes of Hitchcock's need for "participation" in his cinematic world. I elaborate on this "need" by suggesting that, though Hitchcock's corpulence and his generally unconventional appearance foreclosed the possibilities of occupying the dramatic or romantic centers of his films, he still sought validation through performance on the silver screen, however marginal or fleeting. Through his cameos, Hitchcock became *of the screen*, not just the wizard behind it, and thus, received a sort of legitimation that salved the insecurities stemming from his bodily difference from the stars he directed. In short, the Hitchcock cameo is as much a profession of cinematic belonging as virtuosic signature.

When asked about the origin and purpose of his cameos in an interview of the mid-1940s, Hitchcock said:

> It all started with the shortage of extras in my first picture *The Lodger*.[7] I was in for a few seconds as an editor with my back to the camera. It wasn't really much but I played it to the hilt. Since then, I have been trying to get into every one of my pictures which must be 18 or 20 by now. It isn't that I like the business but it has an unholy fascination that I can't resist. When I do, the cast and the grips and the camera men and everyone else for miles around gather to make it as difficult as possible for me. But I can't stop now.[8]

When prompted to speak about the origins of the cameo in interview situations, Hitchcock usually reiterated this same scenario—that, at the time of *The Lodger*, productions were quite small, and that the frame often needed to be filled by faces and bodies; thus the crew (including the director) would assume extra roles, and, therefore, necessity was the mother of the cameo. His daughter Patricia would often tell a similar version of the story in interviews. His evocation of the simpler circumstances of his early films, characterized by modest and makeshift means, and intimacy among cast and crew, is one reason I am drawn to the explanation that his cameo appearances in later films were a ritual that demonstrated homage to and remembrance of his days of filming in England before he became the "Master of Suspense."

Also evident in Hitchcock's recollection of his early cameos is an endearing coyness that partially masks a joy he clearly derives from making an appearance. He tries to establish a reticence through his preemptive remark, "It isn't that I like the business," but he then describes a repulsion-attraction to the idea of performance—in his words, an "unholy fascination" that he "can't stop." His inclusion of the angle of the "cast and the grips and the camera men" colluding to "make it as difficult as possible" bespeaks a sort of hazing, but a kind of loving hazing that at its core confers a sense of belonging. It is this conferral of belonging that the ritualization of the cameo guarantees, from the back of his head in *The Lodger*, to his silhouetted profile in *Family Plot* forty-nine years later. In this chapter, I argue that Hitchcock's cameos are ritual enactments of his belonging to the cinema, a means of consolidating authorial identity, and a vehicle for textual commentary. In what follows, I also perform a close reading of several noteworthy cameo appearances that, in my estimation, mark the films in important ways. I will then put forward a typology of the cameo, explaining certain modes of enunciation in which they operate to install Hitchcock as both auteur and fraternal cinematic performer.

"The Real Me (The Thin One)": Another origin story of the cameo

The story of the origin of the Hitchcock cameo offered above by the man himself was a frequently told tale. He and others would often frame it as a matter of necessity's mothering invention. The need for more extras on a small film set begat the repeated appearance of the director, and he never seemed to "break the habit," even when productions became lavishly populated. When he was honored with the 12th Milestone Award given by the Screen Producers Guild at their awards dinner on March 7, 1965, Hitchcock offered a famously divergent story of the origins of his cameo. The conceit of his after-dinner acceptance speech was, *Who is the real Hitchcock?* In the course of the lighthearted speech, he dismantles four common public misconceptions of the director: that his pictures are harmful in their depiction of violence; that he hates television commercials; that he hates actors, and—most importantly to this chapter—that he is, in fact, fat.

"First of all," Hitchcock jests, "there seems to be a widespread impression that I am stout." Giving the audience time to digest and respond with laughter to this first thread of the appreciative speech, he continues, tongue firmly in cheek: "I can see you share my amusement at this obvious distortion of the truth. Of course I may loom a little large just now, but you must remember, this is before the taxes." Hitchcock presented a variation on this joke ten years earlier in his career, on an *Alfred Hitchcock Presents* introduction, where he sat on one arm of a giant scale, and a pile of moneybags, marked "pounds," filled the other. The joke of the scenario relies on the idea of his being paid by the pound—a visual pun suggesting "pound for pound"—as well as the notion that his size and shape contributed to his celebrity and, consequently, to his fortunes. He makes a similar joke now, equating his weight with his income, which will "slim down" after tax season. He then recalls his first cameo in *The Lodger*, where he was originally to walk up the stairs of the Buntings' rooming house.[9] He continues the joke with sarcasm.

> Since my walk-ons in subsequent pictures would be equally strenuous—boarding buses, playing chess, etc.—I asked for a stunt man. Casting, with an unusual lack of perception, hired this fat man! The rest is history. HE became the public image of Hitchcock. Changing the image was impossible. Therefore I had to conform to the image. It was not easy. But proof of my success is that no one has ever noticed our difference.

The anecdote is delightful and instantly attracted the attention of the press. Herb Stein published a transcript of the speech a week later in the *Morning Telegraph*, in two installments, under the headlines, "Award-Winner Hitchcock Performs Brilliantly," and "Witty Alfred Hitchcock Slays Audience with Barbed Tongue." Ironically, these headlines are two of the few that do not capitalize on his weight, and yet the speech was full of "fat joke" material. Although the story is clearly facetiously intended, this alternative tale of the cameo is telling in its insistence that being fat is not fundamental to his persona, not part of "the real Hitchcock." In this narrative, he only grows fat to match his double ("I had to conform to the image."), thereby re-casting his large size not as a marker of his uncontrolled eating and drinking, but as a sign of his professional commitment to maintaining the illusion of sameness between him and his fictitious "stunt double." In the fantastic and obviously appealing logic of the story, the iconic Hitchcock is not the product of over-eating, but of bad casting.

Hitchcock repeated versions of this story several times; a year after the Screen Producers Guild acceptance speech, he recycled most of the joke while addressing a technical guild, titling the talk, "The Real Me (The Thin One)," hosted, coincidentally, by his old boss in England, Michael Balcon—the employer who had angrily referred to Hitch in the press twenty years earlier as a "plump junior technician." In the different versions of this "Real Me" speech, he typically concluded with the death and re-casting of his stunt double. He would inform the audience that his fat stunt double died tragically, drowning during the filming of *Lifeboat*, because Tallulah Bankhead refused to let him in the boat (and any interference would, of course, have ruined the take). Hitchcock arrives finally at his punch line with this turn of events:

> You may be sure that in securing an actor for my next picture I was more careful. I gave casting an accurate and detailed description of my true self. Casting did an expert job. The result: Cary Grant in *Notorious*. As you know,

> I still remain a prisoner of the old image. They say that inside every fat man is a thin man trying desperately to get out. Now you know that the thin man is the real Alfred Hitchcock.

The last detail is the perfect ending to a great joke, though it cuts to the heart of a poignant concern of this book. As I posit in the introduction, Hitchcock was invested in showing the "real thin man" inside him to his viewing audiences and reading publics. The remarks then are not solely facetious. This narration of the transition from a fat stunt double to Cary Grant as his double is comic, but it also is a barely veiled reference to his dramatic weight loss between *Lifeboat* of 1944 and *Notorious* of 1946. The joke also points to his longstanding idealization of Grant as the perfect male icon of romance and suspense, a relationship I take up in Chapter 5. Thus, the joke is bittersweet. He does, in fact, remain "prisoner of the old image," understanding that the public imagining of Hitchcock will always be that of a fat man, no matter how much his actual body changes. His title "The Real Me (The Thin One)" addresses the joke of the double—a staple figure in his oeuvre, employed in movies such as *Shadow of a Doubt* and *Strangers on a Train*—as well as the confession of his unrequited longing to be seen as a leading man.[10] Hitchcock's fundamental exhibitionist tendencies could never be given free rein, due to his remaining "prisoner of the old image." His cameo appearances, then, mark a compromise between the desire for the cinematic expression of his "true self" and the fat body that rendered this expression impossible.

The (Meso) textual play of the cameo: *Blackmail, Shadow of a Doubt, Lifeboat, Stage Fright*

Having described some of the psychological motivations of the cameo for Hitchcock, in the following, I offer a closer look at how his cameos function in a narrative capacity, using close readings of certain films. I begin by taking a cue from David Sterritt's discussion of the cameo in *Blackmail* (1929). While Sterritt does not commit himself to a full textual and contextual explication of the cameo in *Blackmail*, he lays the groundwork for one, and it is here that I would like to build from his assertion that this particular cameo has "complexities beyond those cited [in his work]."[11] A brief summary of the film will make the significance of the cameo performance much more meaningful.

When the story opens, twenty-something Londoner Alice finds herself in a troubled relationship with Frank, a self-assured policeman. They bicker quite a bit, and Alice has something of a wandering eye. After a tiff in a restaurant, Alice retaliates by going home with an artist named Crewe, who has been eyeing her throughout the altercation. After they drink, collaborate flirtatiously on the drawing of a female nude on a canvas, and then play "dress-up" (Alice changes into a costume at his studio), Crewe becomes violently aggressive in his courtship, and Alice, defending herself and her virtue, stabs him to death. Alice carries the guilty secret alone until Frank, who is assigned to the murder case, finds Alice's glove at the scene of the crime, and realizes her guilt. In addition, a third party, named Tracy, has witnessed the crime and blackmails Alice and Frank. After a confrontation and a chase sequence, Tracy is killed, Frank is able to frame the blackmailer for the murder of Crewe, absolving Alice, and Alice and Frank remain a couple, bound together in their secret knowledge of her guilt.

Hitchcock's cameo occurs ten minutes into the eighty-four-minute film. It is the longest of all of his thirty-nine film appearances, clocking in at nineteen seconds.[12] In it, Hitchcock appears as a passenger on the London Underground.[13] He is seated on the train, occupying the far left hand side of the frame, in medium long shot. To his right are four adults—protagonist Alice, boyfriend Frank, and two other women—and a young boy, seated between the Frank and one of the other women. Immediately, the boy stands up on his seat, looms over Hitchcock, who is guilelessly reading a book (a briefcase beneath the book is also in his lap), and viciously tugs his hat down over his forehead. Hitchcock looks indignant and quickly taps the woman (presumably his mother) on the shoulder, and demands that he be disciplined. The mother shrugs off the complaint, the boy sits down in his seat for a moment, then turns around again, and tugs Frank's hat as well, before hoisting himself up to stare down Hitchcock. Their mutual glare lasts about four seconds, and then the scene dissolves. *Blackmail* was Hitchcock's first sound film (indeed, the first sound film in Britain), and this scene, like many, plays out mostly through pantomime; ambient sounds of the subway absorb most of the characters' speech, though what transpires is clear to the audience. The young child boldly bullies first Hitchcock, and then Frank, and Hitchcock's complaint of being bullied by the child falls on deaf ears.

Aside from the obvious comedy immanent in the scenario, based on the adult Hitchcock's vulnerability at the hands of a small child, the cameo is also a perhaps exaggerated condensation of his own childhood experience of judgment and persecution from peers. As Charlotte Chandler recounts through her interviews with him, Hitchcock's "pudgy, overweight appearance, his lack of interest in the games the other children played, and little athletic ability, isolated him and led to his development of more solitary interior interests." Repeatedly told he was "funny-looking" by disparaging classmates, Hitchcock described himself to Chandler as one of the "homely, less popular children." He confesses, "I found solace in my mother's company, and in my own."[14] Apart from plotting the cameo to riff on his own childhood, Hitchcock also set the stage for an oft-professed antagonism between him and children that would continue to characterize his public persona throughout his career.

Rooting his analysis in the cameo's narrative function, Sterritt observes that the scene depicts a younger, smaller figure who taunts and injures a larger, older character with impunity. He calls this brief interlude a "micro-comedy," the content of which is reflected in the narrative twice after this point. He mentions that a few minutes after this bullying episode, Alice and Frank are at the mercy of a younger and smaller man, a doorkeeper who almost denies them entrance to the restaurant. More importantly, Sterritt remarks that the boy on the subway prefigures the murder of the artist by Alice, another instance of a smaller, younger person wielding power over an older, larger one. Thus, the cameo enacts in miniature a foreshadowing of the murder, in highlighting the conflict chiefly characterized by an age and power differential. While persuaded by the suggestion that Hitchcock's cameo is a "micro-comedy," with facets of foreshadowing, I would suggest that the cameo scene comically prefigures Alice's circumstance, of being victimized without any recourse to, or sympathy from, the patriarchal authority. Instead of viewing the figure of the bullying child as a precursive analogue to Alice later in the film, I contend that the bullied Hitchcock more strongly corresponds to her position after Crewe's death. In other words, the victimized Hitchcock of the cameo better analogizes Alice's position in the murder sequence than the victimizing child.

The difference in this interpretation puts emphasis on different aspects of the power struggle found at the moment of the murder. Sterritt sees the bullying child as analogous to Alice due to her relatively small stature compared to her "victim." Thus, his interpretation focuses on her aggressive act of murder. My interpretation shifts to the victimized status of Alice within the murder scene. The artist clearly intends to rape the unwilling woman; she stabs him in self-defense. The bullying trope, as well as the exploration of the failings of authority figures, are mobilized in other parts of the narrative as well. In addition to the cameo, Sterritt argues that Hitchcock's subjectivity, or at least his sensibility, is represented by several other objects in the film, the main one being the painting of the court jester, now a recognizable icon of early Hitchcock. Sterritt evaluates its presence thusly:

> [The painting of the laughing jester] greets the heroine on her arrival in the room where she will soon (to her own horror) kill a man. The painting

> mutely witnesses this event; later, it hovers in the police station where the killing is being investigated; still later, it punctuates last scene of the story with its silent, sardonic merriment.

Sterritt explains the painting as an exercise in the "Kuleshov effect," whereby it takes on different meanings according to the context in which it is seen. He also calls the painting a "signifier of Hitchcock's control over the narrative and of the shifting (perhaps ambiguous) nature of his own sardonic feelings about the events of the story."[15]

I am more inclined to view the significance of the painting as Tania Modleski does in her essay on *Blackmail* in her wonderful *The Women Who Knew Too Much: Hitchcock and Feminist Theory*. She also views the painting of the jester as a shifting signifier, depending on the context in which it is framed. Yet her emphasis on its shifting signification is slightly different. In tracing the transition of the painting's contextual meanings, she makes the following remarks:

> In the artist's studio Alice at first laughs at the picture and even points back at it, but after she has stabbed Crewe it seems to accuse her, and she lashes out and tears it. Later, when Frank discovers Alice's glove in the studio, he immediately confronts the jester, who appears to be mocking Frank's cuckoldry. At the end, a realignment has clearly taken place, and the sound of male laughter, Frank's included, accompanies the image of the laughing jester pointing at an Alice who can no longer even smile.[16]

While Sterritt focuses on the possibilities of locating the painting as a stand-in for Hitchcock's subjectivity, in his witnessing and commenting on the events of the film, Modleski focuses on the painting as a marker (and bestower) of guilt and of the power dynamics that inhere and diachronically shift in the various transpirations of the plot. Also for Modleski, the painting functions as a screen for the projections of the film's paranoid characters. In the final analysis, Modleski finds that the painting is a "cruel but not unusual joke on woman." As a graphic encapsulation of the accusatory finger and the laughter that surrounds and traps Alice in place, the painting's final meaning in the film is the madness of the patriarchal order that keeps her in a perpetual state of paralysis and silence.

The joke on the woman is multi-layered. Alice is the victim of an attempted rape, but in the eyes of the law, she is a murderer. She has no recourse to the law without being punished as such. Secondly, her boyfriend (with whom she has had lukewarm and unsatisfying relations) is an agent of the law who chooses love over duty and thus does not reveal her guilt when he discovers it. At the end of the film, Alice remains bound to Frank, not of her own volition, but because he retains the knowledge of her guilt which could seal her fate before the law. Modleski connects this truncated female freedom very compellingly with the conclusion of *Marnie* thirty-six years later: "*Blackmail* hints, as *Marnie* will do years later and much more strongly, that the bond linking the man and the woman is his knowledge of her guilty secret (guilty, that is, in patriarchal terms), that the union is founded on the man's ability to blackmail the woman sexually."[17] Thus, through several narrative turns, she becomes the butt of a patriarchal joke by the film's end.

The motif of the unrelenting victimizer and the unaddressed victimized, which, I argue, was presented as tableau in Hitchcock's cameo and then concretized in the uncanny image of the laughing jester, reaches its apotheosis in the denouement. The lack of recourse to authority, posited in the cameo when Hitchcock unsuccessfully appeals to the mother of the offending child to exercise her power and intervene, is echoed in the final scene, when Alice realizes she is outside the law, guilty of patriarchal transgression, and that her recourse to authority in the form of Frank, while preventing literal imprisonment, has occluded any chance for a free life apart from him. Thus, the early Hitchcock cameo sets in motion a foreshadowing of plot, but also a blueprint for the workings of power, knowledge, and gendered authority in the film. While Hitchcock may not take a definitive stance on the irony that characterizes Alice's final circumstances—Modleski finds ambiguity and ambivalence here, where Hitchcock could possibly be celebrating or criticizing the control of women—he is present mesogetically in the film to launch these energizing questions about power and control.[18]

The idea of the Hitchcock cameo as a tableau that sets questions of power and agency in motion can be glimpsed in the very brief appearance of Hitchcock in his beloved 1943 thriller *Shadow of a Doubt*. In this nightmarish tale, teenage Charlie (played by Teresa Wright), discontent with her monotonous and conventional life in suburban Santa Rosa, California, "summons" her uncle and namesake Charlie (played by Joseph Cotten), who comes to visit. The Newton family—Charlie's sister, brother-in-law, nephew and two nieces—is blissfully unaware that Uncle Charlie is in fact the Merry Widow Murderer featured in the newspapers and sought by police in a nationwide manhunt. Young Charlie quickly figures out her uncle's secret identity, and has to reconcile her former idealization of him with the ugly discovery of his misogynist crimes. In addition, she must keep the truth from the police, particularly her new beau, agent Jack Graham, while protecting the family from the awful secret (most importantly, her adoring mother), and must save herself from harm by the ruthless relative. Uncle Charlie is finally killed while attempting to silence Young Charlie, and Charlie and Jack resolve to keep the secret of his crimes so as not to subject the family to devastating disillusionment.[19]

Hitch's cameo in *Shadow* occurs seventeen minutes into the film. In the scene of Hitch's appearance, he is shown on a moving train—the one Uncle Charlie is taking from the East out to Santa Rosa—filmed from behind, holding a bridge hand containing the full suit of Spades, arranged from the 2 to the Ace, left to right. We never see his face, only a medium shot of his back, followed by an extreme close-up on the hand of cards. As the cameo plays out, passengers on the train make inquiries into the health of Charlie, who has secreted himself in his compartment, refusing to see the light of day. Even the porter claims not to have seen the supposedly "very ill" man in question. Critics have remarked that this detail, coupled with our introductory shot of Cotten, where he reclines in bed, shut off from the daylight, gives him a vampiric air, foregrounding his predatory nature and his receiving vitality from the murders of rich women.[20] Charlie's decision to stow himself away, far from the sunlight, perhaps recalls one of Hitchcock's German Expressionist mentors F. W. Murnau, as it resembles Nosferatu's encrypted voyage aboard a rat-infested ship on its way to the fictitious city of Wisborg.

The hand of Spades that Hitchcock holds in the cameo opens a vista of ominous connotations. The Ace of Spades, known as the Death card, and the hand's inclusion of the entire suit of Spades, indicate not only pending death, but as the trump suit in bridge, they may also predict a lethal attack. Soldiers of several twentieth-century wars carried the Ace of Spades card in their helmets or elsewhere on their person into battle as a guarantor of success. Clearly, Uncle Charlie's migration from East to West bodes ill for the Newton family. The card game itself announces a westerly voyage, insofar as the hand of cards partakes of the iconography of the Wild West. The casual card game aboard the train also suggests a game of leisure, chance, and rivalry. The notion of cards as an activity of leisure is resonant in that Charlie's disgust with rich widows is rooted in their frivolous pursuit of leisure on the backs of their hardworking, deceased husbands. Charlie is notably absent from the leisure games of his traveling companions, nestled funereally in his compartment. The hand of Spades also signifies the unpredictable workings of power. Here Hitchcock reminds us that, literally and figuratively, as director, his deck is stacked. The unusual, highly improbable hand suggests having an "upper hand," one that would trump all other hands, yet also carries with it the twinned signifier of precarity and risk; each hand is subject to the luck of the draw. The question of who has the "upper hand" in the film becomes a crucial one, as Uncle Charlie and Charlie relinquish their mutual adoration in becoming absolute adversaries whose wills oppose one another up to the film's climax.

Hitchcock's next film *Lifeboat* (1944), a dramatic portrayal of the erosion of trust, allegiance, and affiliation in the context of the Second World War, posed logistical difficulties for the director's cameo appearance, yet production worked out an ingenious way of insuring his visual presence in the film. In the director's own words, "My easiest assignment from the point of view of performance [in the cameos] was in *Lifeboat*, but at the beginning it looked as though I wouldn't get in at all." *Lifeboat* was one of two Hitchcock films—the other being *Dial M for Murder*—in which he made his cameo in the form of a photograph. Both films posed practical problems for staging a walk-on appearance. The entirety of *Lifeboat* takes place in the middle of the ocean on a rather small vessel, and all of *Dial M for Murder*, apart from the surreal, dystopic moments of Margot Wendice's indictment and conviction by the British court, takes place in the Wendice apartment, as Hitchcock wanted to preserve the unity of space employed in the source play, of the same title, by Frederick Knott. Writers could find no justification for Hitchcock to enter the Wendice apartment, just as they could find no plot device that could account for his presence in the lifeboat. Hitchcock and his writers toyed with the idea of presenting Hitchcock as a corpse that would float by the boat full of survivors.[21] Writers again proposed this floating corpse as a cameo idea almost thirty years later in *Frenzy*, but the strategy was nixed in both films.[22] Hitchcock, in an interview with Charlotte Chandler, recalls feeling tremendously insulted by a joke that resulted from these deliberations. He confides, "What really hurt me was they said I would be just as recognizable floating face-down as face-up. I immediately went on an extreme diet, and that was when I thought of using before-and-after photographs of myself on a page in the newspaper."[23] After ruling out all other means of direct representation, Hitchcock and crew decided upon the indirect—the diegetic photograph.

Twenty-four minutes into the ninety-six-minute film, the camera focuses on the page of a newspaper held by injured passenger Gus (played by William Bendix). Gus relays the article he is reading to his shipmates—a piece that reports the rescue of a group that had been stranded in the ocean for eighty days—and wonders aloud if they would break that record. As he reads, the camera trains on the reverse side of the paper. In the center of the page is a large, eye-catching advertisement for the product *Reduco Obesity Slayer*. Below the product name is a pair of "Before-and-After" photos of Hitchcock standing in what would in time become a familiar profile, facing (his) right. The name "Alfred Hitchcock" is printed beneath the photos, indicating that Hitch is in fact "playing" himself, the famous director, and thereby establishing a link between story and extra-diegetic reality not found in his other cameos. The ad does not reveal what *Reduco* is, but most have assumed it is a diet pill, and Hitchcock, in his interview with Francois Truffaut, confirmed this.

Demonstrating a cameo-induced confusion between diegetic and extra-diegetic reality, audience members reportedly called into Twentieth Century Fox, wondering how to order this wonder drug that had been so successful with the Master of Suspense. Filming late in 1943, Hitchcock was at the end of his first year of relatively successful dieting. While he had not reached his 100-pound goal, he was admirably close to it, and this unconventional cameo became a way for him to exhibit his "new," more streamlined body.

The text of the advertisement reads, "*Reduco* The Sensational New Obesity Slayer. In just 4 months, you too can be slender." The hyperbolic and disingenuous characterization of the ad was an early expression of what would in the 1950s become Hitchcock's well-known contempt for the world of advertising, both televisual and printed. On *Alfred Hitchcock Presents*, he would often take aim at advertisements for being vacuous, dishonest, sensationalistic, and insulting to one's intelligence. In the case of *Reduco*, the notion of "slaying" obesity is a ridiculous and naïve one; more than anyone, Hitchcock knew that obesity could not be "slayed" permanently. The enemy would reappear throughout his life, stronger than ever before. The cameo, then, is a visual joke that scathingly castigates advertisements that play on people's unreasonable expectations.

The cameo is significant for several reasons. Perhaps more than any other, it truly acts mesogetically; it exists as part of the everyday fabric of the story world, and also points clearly outward to Hitchcock's extra-diegetic persona. Not only does the "before-and-after" obviously reference his weight loss in the real world, but it also visually represents his attitude about weight loss. While the "Before" shot captures an obese Hitchcock, he stands erect, gazing out at eye level, in the profile picture. In his "After" photo, he appears quite miserable; his shoulders are hunched and eyes downcast. The difference in Hitchcock's body language in the "before" and "after" is its own subtle joke, perhaps, a commentary on Hitchcock's relationship with food and dieting. In the "after" picture, we have a thinner, sadder Hitchcock, who now understands the stultifying moderation necessary to keep thin, particularly for a middle-aged man experiencing a declining metabolism. What emerges from the cameo is a portrait of a man who once enjoyed the pleasures of consumption and excess, and now is forced to regulate his intake and practice unwelcome self-discipline. Hitch's monumental appreciation for food and drink comes through in this ambivalent rendering—a simultaneous pride in having lost weight and sorrow in forgoing pleasure—which partakes of the fictional and the real equally.

While the camera focuses on the newspaper page for only a brief duration, there is an interesting play of ideas that structure the full composition of the page. One headline on the page reads, "Prominent Citizens, Together With

Civic Bodies, Convene to Make City Park a Success." The headline plays on the word "bodies," referring to the literal body of Hitchcock at the center of the page, and perhaps to the precariously situated bodies on board the lifeboat. Another headline reads, "Fire Destroys State Arsenal," counterbalancing the previous image of building with one of violent undoing. The "arsenal" also references the martial law governing both the world of the film and the world outside. There are also two other ads besides *Reduco* on the page. One reads, "Coats $11;" the other, "Young's FURS. Storage-Remodeling." The contrast evokes class difference, to be sure, and may reflect the disparity of economic status depicted in the relationship between Tallulah Bankhead's wealthy Connie Porter and John Hodiak's working-class John Kovak. In the fashion of typical Hollywood romance, their class difference is first a source of antagonism between the pampered Connie and indignantly proud John, but their romantic attraction belies that initial antagonism. Eventually differences in gender, race, religion, nationality, and beliefs about the goals of war also emerge dramatically to polarize the boat's increasingly desperate passengers, whose bodies are alternately divided in their difference and united in their sameness.

The cameo also makes visible a central thematic concern of the film—the vulnerability of the body. The advertisement heralds the arrival of a product capable of radically altering the body, to give it a more pleasing and acceptable form (the one Hitchcock has always desired). Body modification is a trope germane to the plots of *Lifeboat*. The film begins with the death of a newborn, perhaps the most radical "alteration" of the body. The heavyset Gus, who has been injured in the explosion that caused the nine survivors to scramble for the lifeboat, has his leg amputated, lest the gangrenous infection spread beyond his leg and kill him. Drunkenly he laments the loss of limb, worrying that his sweetheart will not love him anymore because he cannot take her dancing. The characters make frequent reference to injuries they have seen or heard about as a result of the war. Clearly, the war has produced many body modifications, most often gruesome disfigurements caused by landmines, guns, bombs and other *accoutrements* of war. The "Obesity Slayer," offering bodily change that appeals to one's vanity, seems absurd in the context of the epic disfigurations of bodies, troops, and countries that the war has produced. Hitchcock's body stands at the center of this sick joke, trivialized by the gravity of the upheaval surrounding it. More importantly, his cameo in the form of the advertisement provides one of the few, much-needed sources of comic relief, in a drama of disappointment and even despair regarding human nature.

Hitchcock references *Reduco* in his film *Rope* four years later, and it also functions as part of his cameo appearance. We see a brief glimpse of Hitch strolling down the street in the film's opening shot before we move to (and remain in) Brandon and Philip's apartment for the rest of the film. A red neon sign of Hitchcock's famous drawn profile comes to prominence halfway through the film, as the sky darkens. It is an advertisement sign, again for *Reduco*, which is spelled out in neon beneath the profile. The placement of the weight loss advert in view of the apartment is significant, in that the notion of the body-under-surveillance becomes very important in the film. Of course, we spend the film wondering if the body secreted in the trunk will be discovered by the party guests. The boys' maid Mrs. Wilson constantly monitors the guests' consumption. In a maternal pose, she instructs the apparently frail Philip, "You're too thin. Don't let them gobble up the paté before you get to it." Later when the boys' friend Janet Walker, a writer who maintains a column about the "body beautiful," hungrily goes to the buffet (on the trunk), and is immediately checked by Mrs. Wilson, "If I were you, I'd go easy on the paté, dear. Calories." Possibly, these very different reactions on the part of Mrs. Wilson are meant to indicate the cultural tendency to coddle boys (to the point of "spoiling" them) and to deny girls by policing their figure. While the environments of *Lifeboat* and *Rope* are markedly different, the mesogetic intrusion of Hitchcock and *Reduco* may suggest some startling similarities—acts of barbarity, the desperate maintenance of civility in the face of death, the tensions between indulgence and deprivation.

Hitchcock's 1950 film *Stage Fright* marked a return to his native country, his first film based and filmed in England in eleven years. The film tells the story of aspiring young actress Eve Gill (played by American Jane Wyman), who agrees to help fellow actor Jonathan (played by Richard Todd) hide from authorities, who are seeking him for a murder that, he claims, was committed by his lover, glamorous chanteuse Charlotte Inwood (Marlene Dietrich). Eve not only harbors the fugitive, but goes "undercover," posing as a working-class dresser in order to get proof of Charlotte's guilt and thereby exonerate Jonathan. In the course of her own investigation, she crosses paths with Detective Wilfred Smith, assigned to the murder case, much like Jack Graham in *Shadow*. In the end, Eve discovers that her friend Jonathan is actually guilty of the murder, and she narrowly escapes being murdered by him. In the conclusion, Eve is saved, Jonathan dies, and Wilfred Smith becomes Eve's new love interest.

Of his thirty-nine cameo appearances, only four depict any interaction between Hitchcock and a main character.[24] None of these interactions is verbal.[25] In *Marnie* (1964), Hitchcock enters a corridor of a hotel just after Tippi Hedren's Marnie has passed by, and he fixes his gaze on her as she enters her room, before casting his eye toward the camera knowingly. As discussed in Chapter 2, Hitchcock and the songwriter exchange a few unintelligible words as he winds the clock in his apartment in *Rear Window*. Cary Grant eyes Hitch somewhat suspiciously as they sit next to each other on a bus in *To Catch a Thief* (1955). And finally, thirty-nine minutes into the 110-minute *Stage Fright*, Hitchcock passes Jane Wyman's Eve Gill, and then stops, turns around to regard her, as she is in disguise, practicing her Cockney-inflected introduction to diva Charlotte Inwood, rehearsing the role of her alter ego, "Doris Tinsdale." Comically, Hitchcock casts her a withering look of disbelief, then exits the frame. Hitchcock spoke to the *New York Times* on June 4, 1950 and discussed this particular cameo.

> I have been told that my performance is quite juicy; I have been told this with a certain air of tolerance, implying that I have now achieved the maximum limits of directorial ham in the movie sandwich. It isn't true. There may have been a "MacGuffin" in my film appearance, but not a ham.[26]

No doubt, there is a certain cheekiness in Hitchcock's appearance in *Stage Fright*; it is perhaps the only one of the thirty-nine that captures Hitchcock in the act of judging one of his main characters. This moment of the cameo, when Eve is practicing the speech and mannerisms of her alter ego, the persona through which she is investigating the murder by trying to secure proof of Charlotte Inwood's guilt, is but one of quite a few that emphasize the importance of acting and disguise to the film. In this regard, *Stage Fright* may be regarded as an embryonic form of exploration so expertly executed by *Rear Window* four years later, deploying theatricality and performance as meta-tropes, meant to underscore a kind of self-referentiality about cinema and its illusions.

The scenario of playacting also reinforces one of Hitchcock's major themes—that of appearance versus reality, coupled with the notion that everyone plays roles more or less convincingly, and that success largely depends on inhabiting roles of great artifice.[27] No one is "natural," *per se*. Locating the action in the world of the theater helps to convey the ubiquitous signifiers of performativity. In trying to transform herself, Eve has affected a thoroughly unconvincing Cockney accent, belied by her genteel upbringing, and even her cheap clothes and newly acquired habit of smoking do not convincingly disguise her. Just prior to the cameo, she rings her own doorbell, and her mother, upon answering, recognizes Eve immediately and does not even comment on her attempt at disguise.

In this instance, it is safe to assume that Hitchcock performs as a spectator surrogate in his cameo role. His disbelief in her "Doris Tinsdale" persona echoes our own disbelief that a sheltered and refined girl could pass as a cousin of the rough Nellie Bly. Her performance has failed on every level, and for every audience, inside and outside the film, and Hitchcock's gaze of disbelief cements that failure. In terms of story, this disbelief shared by mother, Hitchcock, and audience, in addition to its comedy, also creates a suspenseful sense of trepidation, as we wonder how on earth Eve can convince Charlotte Inwood of her disguise. As luck would have it, Charlotte is so self-absorbed, she does not pay enough attention to Eve to notice that the performance is a very poor one; the only one that matters to her is her own. Hitchcock's cameo may also be a gentle wink at the notion that Wyman was one of the only Americans in the almost entirely British cast. Thus, the cameo links the diegetic concern of a character's "passing" with the extra-diegetic matter of Wyman's affecting an accent not her own.

Hitchcock's disbelief at Eve's poor portrayal of a working-class girl may also mimic our own disbelief at Hitchcock's appearance in the film. The cameos are always slightly surreal, as they effect a momentary narrative confusion. In my argument for the term "mesogesis," I refrain from characterizing Hitchcock's appearance as a total rupture of the diegetic world, but it certainly stretches the diegesis outward, toward the real, as we note the uncanny parallelism of the extra-diegetic with the established filmic reality we have come to accept. Therefore, Eve's inadequate performance as "Doris" may occasion an appraisal of our own responses to Hitchcock-the-director's transition into Hitchcock-the-actor/character. In this performance of skepticism, Hitchcock perhaps lets us know that he is "in on the joke." His appearance is "unnatural," just like most participants in the world of *Stage Fright*. The notion of "stage fright," performance anxiety, seems to be an alien fear to Hitchcock, the avowed exhibitionist. Thus, this sense of play established with the idea of theatricality and performance works on several levels; Hitchcock is begging our pardon for the unconventional nature of his appearances. They are a compulsion for him, an "unholy fascination," that reveals the depths of his love for show business and his desire to inhabit both sides of the camera.

A typology of the Hitchcock cameo

The thirty-nine cameo appearances of Hitchcock's career (that made it to the released film) cannot all fit neatly into discrete categories, in terms of their nature, effect, or narrative function, though there are several compelling repetitions and consistencies that emerge when they are regarded *in toto*.[28] The most common of these is the cameo of *Hitchcock in Transit*. There are nineteen appearances of a traveling Hitchcock, eight of which are on foot (*Easy Virtue*, *Rebecca*, *I Confess*, *The Trouble With Harry*), and eleven at locations of mass transit, either on, in, or near vehicles: at Victoria Station in *The Lady Vanishes*; on a bus in *Number 17* and *To Catch a Thief*; missing a bus in *North*

By Northwest; on a subway in *Blackmail*; boarding, unboarding or riding a train in *Strangers on a Train*, *The Paradine Case*, and *Shadow of a Doubt*; in a wheelchair at an airport in *Topaz*; getting off an elevator in *Spellbound*.

It is not surprising to find that many of Hitchcock's cameos occur in scenarios of travel and mass transit. It is, of course, in travel that many of Hitchcock's characters become entangled in the dramatic situations of his films. In travel, identities are in flux; his characters frequently take opportunities to slough their pasts and reinvent themselves, whether brunette Mary Rogers becomes blonde Marnie Edgar, Marion Crane checks in to a motel as Marie Samuels, or Roger Thornhill gives instructions to a valet as George Kaplan. Relationships made while traveling are often temporary, usually utilitarian, and frequently cloaked in deceit. Thus, his cameo placement in sites of travel indicates his imaginative investment—and his audiences', as well—in narratives of palpable flux, fantastic transition, re-fashioned identity—in short, the stories of identification and desire that constitute the visual pleasure of his films.

In five of his films, Hitchcock appears in crowd scenes, as a spectator. *Hitchcock the Spectator* is present for a moment in the lynch mob in pursuit of the Avenger in *The Lodger*; he holds a camera outside the courthouse in *Young and Innocent*; in *Under Capricorn*, he appears first in the town square during a parade, and ten minutes later on the steps of a government building; he watches a performance of acrobats in the marketplace in the 1956 version of *The Man Who Knew Too Much*; and finally, in *Frenzy*, he is part of an audience listening to a political speaker, and then a minute later, among the onlookers watching as a victim of the Necktie Strangler has been found floating in the Thames.

The occasions for spectatorship of these cameos range from the civic-minded, to the commercial, to the prurient. Most obviously, Hitchcock as crowd participant evokes the parallels of his spectatorship with ours, the audience. In this sense, we may be led to consider these moments as ones of viewer surrogacy, where the director stands in for us in our specular curiosity and engagement. And the varying contexts—the political speech, the media spectacle, the exposed dead woman—run the gamut of our specular investments, whether we watch for pleasure, information, or simply because everyone else is. In this regard, Hitchcock the gawker may be extending an ethical hand to his audience: *I watch for the reasons you watch*; *my pleasure is your pleasure*; *my curiosity is your curiosity.* The cameos also mark the crowd scenes with a moment of mesogetic irony, as the sight of the spectating Hitchcock creates a pleasurable dissonance with our knowledge that he has in fact orchestrated every situation, environment, and interaction of the film.

Hitchcock may also be using these moments of the spectator-cameo to make more localized, film-specific comments. In *The Lodger*, he appears both at the editorial desk of the newspaper, and then in the angry mob intent on catching the (wrong) killer. Taken together, we may note that one of his appearances is in the ostensibly neutral space of the media, where he is responsible for level-headed reportage; in the next, he is absorbed by a mob's mentality, hell-bent on misplaced vengeance. The two considered in concert may suggest the media's responsibility for generating conflagrations and public sentiment without adequate knowledge of the facts. In his *Frenzy* cameo, Hitchcock, long influenced by the cognitive insights of Soviet Montage, instructively evokes the Kuleshov Effect. The notion that the meanings of images change based on context—suggested earlier in my response to Sterritt's discussion of *Blackmail*—is given wicked illustration, when Hitchcock first gazes at a politician and then, moments later, gazes at a strangled woman. Based on the object of the gaze, we perceive Hitch's look quite differently. The parallelism of *Hitchcock the Spectator*'s gaze in these two scenarios may also suggest that the politician (whom Hitchcock is the sole spectator *not* to applaud) is no less mired in the sordid than the surfacing nude corpse.

A third category of cameo is one that I have mentioned earlier in my discussion of *Stage Fright*: *Hitchcock as Character*. In proposing this category, I do not mean to imply that these are the only moments he functions as a diegetic character, but that, due to his proximity to characters who are vital to the narrative, he appears to us closer to the heart of the story, more anchored in the filmic reality than *Hitchcock the Spectator* or *Hitchcock in Transit*. Hitchcock's decision to appear in the same frame as his lead actors represents, perhaps, an intensification of the desire for the "conferral of belonging" to the cinema that I have evoked early in this chapter.

There are four such instances: *Rear Window* (discussed at length in Chapter 2); the aforementioned *Stage Fright*; *To Catch a Thief*; and finally, *Marnie*. In *Rear Window*, Hitchcock appears in the apartment of the songwriter, winding a clock on the mantle while conversing with the composer as he sits at his piano.[29] Hitchcock's winding of the clock in the cameo points to the importance of temporality to the film, especially as the notion of time and change are ones to which Jefferies is particularly resistant at the opening of the film. He prefers the fantasy of a static world and eroticizes the static image, yet Hitchcock as director and character wields the clock to remind us that time cannot stand still. In *To Catch a Thief*, Hitchcock appears on a bus, sitting next to his lead actor Cary Grant. The cameo is particularly funny as a mesogetic moment, in its pointing to the extra-filmic reality of the relationship between Hitchcock and Grant. In the cameo, Grant eyes Hitchcock somewhat suspiciously. This casual slight is humorously at odds with the director's love and admiration for the actor in real life. Hitchcock has famously been quoted as revealing, "Cary Grant is the only actor I ever loved." Hitchcock's relationship with Grant is characterized both by identification and desire (which I will examine at length in Chapter 6). Thus, the cameo relies on our extratextual knowledge of this relationship for its humor, in foregrounding the very different nature of reality within and outside the story world of *To Catch a Thief*.

In *Marnie*, one of Hitchcock's later films, Hitchcock appears in a hotel corridor at the very beginning of the film, just as Marnie walks past with a valet and enters her own room. This appearance marks the only cameo placement in which Hitchcock actually breaks the cinematic fourth wall. As mentioned earlier, after gazing at Tippi Hedren's character for a moment, he then directs his eyes to the camera, giving it/us a knowing look. Not only does this moment suggest that Marnie is recurrently the object of the gaze in the film, but it also introduces her as an object of suspicion. In her life as a thief, she relies on changing her appearance to avoid capture, and even before we know this about her character, Hitchcock appears to single her out, to let us know that this is a woman to be watched. It may also forge a tacit connection to his walk-on in *Stage Fright*; in both situations, Hitchcock the observer is not buying the act of the disguised woman he watches. In this manner, Hitchcock's insight into Marnie prefigures Mark's (Sean Connery).

The fourth category of cameo that emerges from considering all of films together is *Hitchcock as Virtuoso*. In four different films, all between 1945 and 1958, Hitchcock walks into his cameo carrying an instrument case: a violin in *Spellbound*; a cello in *The Paradine Case*; a double bass in *Strangers on a Train*; and a trumpet (or bugle) in *Vertigo*.[30] The instrument motif is in line with several comments Hitchcock made throughout his career concerning the orchestration of suspense and his manipulation of the audience. He famously quipped, "I like to play the audience like a piano."[31] In a publicity piece for *Psycho*, he stands in a theater lobby outside a packed house watching his most famous horror film, and as an orchestral conductor, he "conducts" the screams and wails of terror that emanate from the theater as the shower scene plays in front of them. We never see Hitchcock play the piano in the frames of his films, though we watch see him carrying three woodwind instruments and one brass. The idea of Hitchcock's "playing the audience" like an instrument is interesting in the context of a cameo appearance, where any other director would likely efface any reference to his own orchestrations and manipulations of plot and character. Of course, Hitchcock does not play by the rules; his decision to highlight his own status as master manipulator—as conductor and player—only makes the moment more—for lack of a better word—*Hitchcockian*.

The signification of the individual instruments Hitchcock carries may offer some insight into their purpose, connecting the cameo with the finer workings of the world of the story. The violin may be appropriate to *Spellbound* as the Bergman-Peck romance is so firmly foregrounded in the film, the violin's associations with romance and drama become clear. The cello of *The Paradine Case* is a lower, often darker variation on the violin, and of course, the story of the film is much darker; love is nothing to celebrate in this film, as it is in *Spellbound.* The double bass of *Strangers on a Train* represents the lowest tonal register of the string family. In his cameo, Hitchcock struggles with the largest and most physically cumbersome of the string instruments. Several critics have noticed that the shape of the double bass is used as a comic commentary on Hitchcock's physique, that the bottom-heavy instrument is a sort of visual Hitchcockian double, in a film that depends so much for its intrigue and its exploration of identity through the form of the double.[32]

Vertigo is the last of his films to use an instrument prop in the cameo, and in it Hitchcock has moved to the brass family. Because the trumpet and bugle are used for playing *Taps* and *Last Rites* in military funerals, Hitchcock's wielding of the instrument, just before Scottie meets Elster and becomes entangled with the funereal Madeleine, seems particularly, and eerily, appropriate. Arriving eleven minutes into the film, we watch Hitchcock cross the screen with the trumpet/bugle case, just as Scottie is entering the offices of villain Gavin Elster. Norman Holland describes the cameo's significance as the announcement of a fundamental diegetic transition.

> He walks across the film frame, carrying a trumpet case, as Scottie is about to go upstairs to Elster's office in the shipyard. I read Hitchcock as marking the move from one world to another. He is a Pied Piper, leading Scottie away from the realistic world. . . . [Scottie] enters the mysterious world that Elster will build for him.[33]

Clearly, there are many Hitchcock films that do not fit neatly into the aforementioned categories. Hitchcock does not seem to have had any kind of overarching plan for the cameos, which spanned from 1927 to 1976. I have merely gathered certain repetitions or similarities that appear from time to time without proposing a definitive schematic. In three cameos, Hitchcock is smoking a cigarette; in three, he reads a newspaper. Nine cameos present "comic" scenarios.[34] In five cameos, Hitchcock is fully stationary; two involve children; three contain animals; three use his silhouette; one shows him drinking; another shows him littering. Nothing unites them beyond their iconicity as film-events that audiences grew to cherish over time.

In my earlier analysis of the cameo of *Stage Fright*, I suggested that Hitchcock's comic skepticism regarding Eve Gill's performance of the role "Doris Tinsdale" might occasion our own sense of being comically wary of Hitchcock's textual presence as "not convincing" in itself. If Eve's unconvincing portrayal of Doris leads us to think about Hitchcock's presence as "unconvincing," what would that mean? Of what do we as an audience need to be convinced? Are we to be convinced that, in the director's appearance in the mesogetic space opened up by the cameo, that the filmic world parallels or is convincingly analogous to our world? Does the cameo simply affirm that the filmic world is entirely of Hitchcock's making? Is the cameo an invitation to partake of the filmic world like Hitchcock mischievously has done, imaginatively inserting ourselves into the world of the story? Is he performing in the capacity of creator, bystander, chorus, translator, the great Enunciator or just a working actor?

Hitchcock's visual and dramatic participation in the filmic world of his construction, however brief and fleeting, had its own gratifications that we may never fully understand. In divining the pleasure with which he often spoke about his cameos, I am convinced that these appearances were therapeutic, beyond their narrative functions. Hitchcock was confident enough in his craft that he required little external acknowledgment of his cinematic mastery. The cameos, however, provided a different kind of acknowledgment; they constituted proof of his belonging, not just with his cast and crew, not just with the characters he created and realized, but also with the world of cinematic visibility. Cameos rendered Hitchcock's body cinematic; throughout his career, they continued to offer an affirmation that flew in the face of the conventional wisdom that his fatness should exclude him from the stringent and unforgiving visual economy of Hollywood productions. Hitchcock created and nurtured the tradition of the cameo that honored his filmmaking from its beginnings, and celebrated his own filmic possibilities from within and outside of his productions.

3

The pleasures and pangs of Hitchcockian consumption

People say, "Why don't you make more costume pictures?" Nobody in a costume picture ever goes to the toilet. That means, it's not possible to get any detail into it. People say, "Why don't you make a western?" My answer is, I don't know how much a loaf of bread costs in a western. I've never seen anybody buy chaps or being measured or buying a 10 gallon hat. This is sometimes where the drama comes from for me.[1]

By 1942, Hitchcock had acquired his legendary moniker the "Master of Suspense." The nickname proved more accurate and durable than the title David O. Selznick had tried to confer on him—"the Master of Melodrama"—a year earlier, after *Rebecca*'s release. In a fifty-four-feature career, he deviated only occasionally from his tried and true suspense film, with the exceptions of his early British assignments, the horror films *Psycho* and *The Birds*, the splendid, darkly comic *The Trouble with Harry*, and the romantic comedy *Mr. and Mrs. Smith* of 1941, which he is said to have made purely out of loyalty to friend Carole Lombard. When asked why he did not branch out into other genres, Hitchcock generally replied with some variation on the reply he gave Fletcher Markle above on his TV show *Telescope*.

The elliptical explanation he was known to offer—"Nobody in a costume picture ever goes to the toilet," and "I don't know how much a loaf of bread costs in a western"—should tell us several things. First, it points to a particular ethos of verisimilitude in representation for which critics have applauded him throughout his film career—his careful attention to detail within the mise-en-scene of his films. Hitchcock assiduously avoided anachronism, left nothing extraneous, nothing without visual explanatory power, in his frame, and was wholly and consistently devoted to a realism that governed the life of objects and people in his films. It points to Hitchcock's need to know the ins and outs of the material world of his film, including the small transactions, before he could begin to realize a drama within it.

It is also quite telling that Hitchcock (repeatedly) offered the examples that he did. His microscopic focus on human habits, behaviors, and obligations such as going to the toilet and buying bread are, for him, benchmarks of that commitment to realism. They reveal his belief in grounding his cinema in the banal, the quotidian, the material realities and exchanges of human existence that often receive representational short shrift in the cinema of other directors. These small moments of transaction, he says, are "sometimes where the drama comes from."

Of course, food and drink were incredibly important both in the director's own personal life, as well as in his motion pictures. Food was not just sustenance for Hitchcock; it was inspiration, fantasy, a window to sublimity. As he once told a reporter in New York, "There is as much anticipation in confronting good food as there is in going on a holiday or seeing a good show. There are two kinds of eating—eating to sustain and eating for pleasure. I eat for pleasure." When Hitchcock hired new actors and writers for his productions, he most often used conversations about food and drink to break the ice with them, whether it was how to prepare batter pudding with *Frenzy*'s Anna Massey; how to find good wine in Bristol, with (twelve-year-old) Veronica Cartwright of *The Birds*; how donuts are made, with Tippi Hedren; or how to make pork cracklings, with writer David Freeman. For Hitchcock, friendship bonding happened over food and drink. A sure sign of his acceptance was an invitation to his always plentiful dinner table.

In what follows, I explore the various ends to which Hitchcock deployed food and drink beyond the sustenance of a realist aesthetic. Specifically, I locate moments when he grounds food and drink in philosophical inquiries about the relationship between pleasure and disgust (the polarized ambivalence which characterized his own consumption of food and drink); further, I examine his use of processes of consumption and elimination to dramatize sublimation, particularly sexual sublimation; to explore the nature of his characters' vulnerabilities; to metaphorize the narrative flow of information and the nature of his characters' interactions; and to convey particular attitudes toward his characters. We will begin with the status of the body in Hitchcock's films.

Screening the revolting body

The pleasure and disgust that alternately governed Hitchcock's feelings about food and drink similarly describe his attitudes toward the human body and its capacities for consumption and elimination. As much as he framed the body as a source of scopic pleasure in his films, he also frequently directed our cinematic gaze to the body as a site of abjection, and exploited it as such, albeit less frequently and less explicitly in his filmmaking than in his life off screen. Throughout his career, Hitchcock retained a self-confessed puerile sense of humor rooted in the functions of the body, which for him were endlessly funny and bizarre. He would often use a whoopie cushion on new guests to his house, and would feign horror and dismay as the unsuspecting guest sat on the flatulent toy.[2] He seemed to enjoy the incommensurability of the dignified English gentleman's persona he performed in public, with the private jokester who could not help but titter at the mention of unmentionables.

In the late 1920s, he laid a bet with one of his cameramen that the latter could not spend a night in the supposedly haunted film studio, chained to his camera. The unwitting man accepted the bet, as well as a carafe of brandy, courtesy of Hitchcock, that had been spiked with laxatives, to get him through the night. The next day, the crew arrived to find the mortified winner of the bet, who had ruined his pants in the process—a sight that delighted the director. A running joke in several of his films involved his use of the initials B. M. (an abbreviation for "bowel movement"): characters Bob Marvin in *The Secret Agent* (1936), Barbara Morton in *Strangers on a Train* (1951), Ben McKenna in *The Man Who Knew Too Much*, and Babs Milligan and Brenda Margaret Blaney in *Frenzy* (1972). Additionally, John Hodiak displays a chest tattoo of the initials in *Lifeboat* (1944), and the "engagement" ring of *Shadow of a Doubt* bears the inscription "TS, from BM."

It was common for him to introduce himself jokingly (to men, rarely to women), as "Hitch, without the *cock*." This is, of course, a crude joke, but it also points to a biographical fact that Hitchcock did not mind sharing in some intimate company: his lack of sexual experience and his impotence throughout most of his adult life. During the shooting of *The Birds*, he described himself as "long chaste," and either joked or confessed that he had had proper sex only once, to father his daughter Patricia. Several times, to the chagrin of Alma and in the presence of friends, he would share, regarding his size at the time of Pat's conception, "I was so fat I had to conceive my daughter with a fountain pen!"[3]

Clearly, elements of Hitchcock's lifestyle during most of his time as an adult—such as his weight, poor circulation from sedentary work days, and heavy drinking—conspired to challenge his sexual performance. Hitchcock's lack of bedroom experience, however, evidently did not curb his interest in bodies, sex, and sexuality—quite the opposite. His sexual dysfunction, though, may shed some light on the importance for him of rendering the body, its processes and its irregularities, comically. In another context, he candidly confessed to Francois Truffaut, "I'm a celibate, you know. I'm not against it, but I don't think about it very much."[4] This cinematic focus on the absurd and unpredictable aspects of embodiment offered a way for him to avoid the pitfalls of idealizing the life of physicality that was unavailable to him. To his immense credit and to our benefit, Hitchcock chose to see his sexual outsider status as conducive to the creative process, rather than detrimental. To friend Charlotte Chandler, he said:

> I think that too much sex while you are working goes against the work and that repressed sex is more constructive for the creative person. It must get out, and so it goes into the work. I think it helped create a sense of sex in my work. The experiencing of passion, as with fear, makes you feel alive. In the film, you can experience these very extreme feelings without paying the bill.

While this rationalization may employ a reductive or overly simplistic account of sublimation and the channeling of desire, it doubtless expresses Hitchcock's attitudes about cinema as an outlet for desire, both on the part of creator and spectator. Hitchcock proves time and again that cinema was not just a space to glorify the body beautiful; it was a medium in which we could glimpse the comic and dramatic facets of our body's vulnerabilities and occasional embarrassments.

One particular preoccupation with the body and its lower functions can be glimpsed in the frequency with which Hitchcock conceived scenes that portrayed his lead characters in the throes of nausea. The visual depiction of vomiting was never directly addressed in the Production Code of 1930s Hollywood, though it may arguably have been covered in the code's statements about vulgarity in Section III: "The treatment of low, disgusting, unpleasant, though not necessarily evil, subjects should be guided always by the dictates of good taste and a proper regard for the sensibilities of the audience."[5] Because there were no such restrictions in place for films produced in England at the time, Hitchcock felt free to show his two leads Fred and Emily vomiting in his 1931 British film *Rich and Strange* with impunity. The scene was comedic in tone; the husband and wife (played by Henry Kendall and Joan Barry) vomit over the side of a boat after discovering that they have consumed cat meat in their last meal.

However, when Hitch arrived in America, the Hays Code had been in effect since 1933, under the watchful eye of Joseph Breen.[6] Despite the code's articulation of "disgusting, unpleasant subjects," which would seem to occlude the presentation of characters vomiting, Hitchcock tried several times to include such scenarios. In his first American production *Rebecca*, he supervised a treatment that contained two scenes of characters vomiting which David O. Selznick, his producer, immediately pronounced unfilmable. In the initial treatment of an opening scene coauthored by Hitchcock and Alma, several passengers aboard a boat to Monte Carlo are made ill by the lead Maxim's (Laurence Olivier) cigar smoke. Several scenes later, in this same treatment, the protagonist, the second Mrs. De Winter (known in the script as "I" and called "Daphne" by Selznick and crew) embarrasses herself by vomiting from a combination of nerves and seasickness. Selznick was outraged at the representation, and sent it back to Hitchcock swimming in red ink. He ordered many changes, including the striking of the scenes of nausea, with the final word on the matter: Women do not vomit in Hollywood.

The issue resurfaced five years later, this time without the censorial intrusions of strong-willed Selznick, as Hitchcock and collaborator Ben Hecht were finalizing the script for *Notorious*, they struggled to come up with a satisfactory ending, and in the process produced pages with very different conclusions. In one discarded version, Ingrid Bergman's Alicia dies in Cary Grant's arms while being rescued from the clutches of Alex Sebastian (played by Claude Rains) and his mother (Leopoldine Konstantin). The script concludes back in Miami, where Grant's Devlin sits in a café alone with his memory of Alicia, trying to remain stoic while he listens to bystanders malign her. In a second draft—the final scenes of which were authored by Hitchcock—Devlin rescues Alicia successfully, and as they escape from the Sebastian mansion, she vomits all over the front steps.[7] The image of Alicia's nausea dissolves into the film's resolution: they have returned to Miami, where Alicia is pardoned for her connections with the Nazi party, and she and Devlin are married by the Justice of the Peace. Obviously, the final shooting script takes the middle road, resorting neither to Alicia's (explicit) death nor to the couple's marriage; it also omits Alicia's vomiting upon her rescue.[8]

The decision to remove the vomiting scene may have been made in deference to the Hays Code, or as a simple concession to good taste. I would argue that the inclusion of Alicia's nausea in these final moments may have in fact rendered the film's conclusion more Hitchcockian. As it stands, Devlin's heroic rescue is atypically idealized for a Hitchcock ending. Bergman here is filmed with a gauzy, ethereal light, making her look soft and beautiful even in her profound sickness. Donald Spoto, in his analysis of *Notorious*, characterizes the reunion of Alicia and Devlin as "perhaps the tenderest, truest love scene in his entire filmography. It's straight from the pages of a fairy tale—Prince Not-So-Charming Awakens Snow-Beige."[9] The inclusion of the scene of nausea would perhaps have been a corrective to this visual idealization, more in keeping with Hitchcock's aesthetic and narrative sensibilities, endowing it with an earthier sense of realism and a greater sense of ambivalence about both the rescue and the prospects of the romantic relationship. Filming Alicia's nausea would have militated against her being read as an angelic figure, a characterization that is not at all consistent with her portrayal as a promiscuous alcoholic established from the film's opening frames. Her vomiting would also have provided a potent visual resolution to the central trope of intoxication (encapsulating both Alicia's drinking problem and the Sebastians' conspiracy to poison her slowly) that threads through *Notorious*. The decision to forgo the shots of Alicia's nausea results in a more hygienic, more contained, ending than that to which the Hitchcock spectator is accustomed (thus, Spoto's enthusiastic claims for the film's romance). The only truly Hitchcockian ambiguity resides in the refusal to screen Alicia's ultimate fate.

In addition to these scenes of nausea in *Rebecca* and *Notorious* that never saw the light of day, several other Hitchcock films implicitly suggest the vomiting of female characters. In *The Birds* (1963), as Melanie and the Brenner family await the final onslaught of the film's climax, young Cathy intriguingly turns to Melanie the family outsider, crying, "Melanie! Melanie, I'm going to be sick!" The moment is interesting, particularly as Cathy turns to Melanie, the woman who has threatened to overtake Lydia's maternal role, for comfort. If, as much criticism suggests, the final attack on Melanie is a moment that transforms her into a child—helpless, inchoate, all-fearful—this moment of Cathy's nausea which precedes the attack may, in fact, be read as the onset of menstruation. The shuffling of the permutations of the nuclear family structure that constitutes the shifting Oedipal triangulation of the film perhaps requires that Cathy abandon the child position through physical maturation, leaving Melanie as the powerless child over whom Lydia has maternal dominion. The suggestion of nausea as a signifier of the arrival of menstruation here opens up a fascinating vista revealing how power, sexuality, and maternity are connected in the schema of Hitchcock's Bodega Bay.

In *Dial M for Murder* (1954), murder committed in self-defense is the occasion for a woman's nausea. Upon turning on the lights and realizing that she has killed Lesgate (Anthony Dawson) in self-defense, Margot (Grace Kelly) covers her mouth in horror, stumbles to the bedroom, pauses at the door while clutching her stomach, and then heads for the bathroom. The scene dissolves to a panicked Margot's greeting her husband (Ray Milland) at the front door of the apartment. In this case, nausea would be a dramatically justified, realistic response to an accidental murder. Hitchcock's 1972 *Frenzy*, a film that is shot through with allusions to, and images of, trash, waste, filth, and abjection, also depicts the implicit suggestion of a woman's vomiting. In this instance, however, the nausea plays as comic relief: Chief Inspector Oxford, who has been subjected to his wife's forays into the more adventurous side of French cuisine, retaliates against her near the end of the film, insulting her culinary failures, after holding his tongue throughout several unpalatable dinners. When Mrs. Oxford suggests that it would be appropriate to invite the wrongly incarcerated Blaney over for a conciliatory dinner, her husband retorts, "After that jail food he's been having, I suspect he'll eat anything." Affronted, she downs the salt-rimmed margarita she had earlier prepared for Sergeant Spearman, and subsequently makes a hasty retreat to the kitchen. Looking green around the gills, she grabs her stomach, and exits the frame, feebly mumbling, "Excuse me, I must see if my soufflé has started to rise." Her exit line's comedic effect draws from the substitution of Mrs. Oxford's rising soufflé for her rising bile.

Hitchcock again employs nausea in his final film *Family Plot*, and again, he exploits the figure of the nauseated woman to comic effect. Blanche, the charlatan clairvoyante (played with verve by Barbara Harris), is portrayed as vivacious, headstrong, and lusty; this characterization comes through in part through the depiction of her hearty appetites, both culinary and sexual. After energetically devouring one hamburger, she orders her partner George (played by Bruce Dern) to make her another. He denies her request ("You don't need another one; you already got one."), and hurries her to the car, where shortly thereafter they become involved in a car chase. As Blanche and George wind their way through the Hollywood hills at top speed, Blanche cautions George to slow down, screaming out, "My hamburger is coming up again!" The allusion to vomiting caps off the slapstick of the car chase—a scene that, according to Dern, made Hitchcock laugh hysterically during its filming.

This recurring depiction of nausea demonstrates Hitchcock's desire to capture the body even, and sometimes especially, in its moments of unsavory weakness. It is interesting to consider why six of his seven characters that experience nausea are female. To write this off as simple misogyny is to preclude more interesting discoveries about Hitchcock's relationship to gender and embodiment. The answer may lie in part in an early interview conducted by Barbara Buchanan in a 1935 article provocatively entitled, "Alfred Hitchcock Tells a Woman that Women Are a Nuisance." The interview begins by reporting Hitchcock's frustration with English actresses, most pointedly in their refusal to relinquish their "ladylike" postures on camera. He explains:

> If I were directing Claudette Colbert (whom I consider to be one of the loveliest women in American film), I should first show her as a mannequin.

> She would slink through the showroom, in her elegant French way, wearing gorgeous gowns as only such a woman can. . . . Then I should show her backstage. As she disappeared through the curtains, I'd make her suck down a piece of toffee or chewing gum which she had kept in her mouth all the time she was looking so beautiful—you see what I mean? That touch of realism would make her infinitely more human.[10]

Hitchcock characterizes the idealization of the female figure as a detriment to a woman's cinematic performance, as well as to a film's sense of realism. He continues, "It is always their desire to appear a lady and, in doing so, they become cold and lifeless. Nothing pleases me more than to knock the ladylikeness out of chorus girls! I try to make a woman human by making her appear in awkward and comic situations and taking away her glamour."[11] In this optic, the motive for inflicting nausea upon his female characters seems rooted in this nod to realism and the belief that women need to be called back to a less mediated, less self-conscious body as a means of militating against the sort of idealization that renders them inaccessible to film audiences. One wonders if there is not a degree of schadenfreude attached to the motive for taking his female stars down a notch. His longstanding frustration with women he perceived as romantically inaccessible may find a perverse satisfaction in staging their humiliation through these scenes of nausea, both in comic and dramatic situations.

In sussing out the factors that compelled Hitchcock to make (specifically female) nausea a source of dramatic expression and comedic release, it is also important to understand that, according to Spoto, Hitchcock as a child had been terrified of vomiting.[12] For him, vomiting signified a disturbing loss of bodily control. When Hitch had been performing as assistant director in Germany in 1923–24, he began to experience extreme nausea, not due to anything toxic he consumed, but out of a sense of social claustrophobia he experienced being in a foreign land surrounded by workers who knew little English. This fear of losing bodily control is consistent with Hitchcock's obsessive need for order and transparency in his home and work environments. Perhaps, then, these moments of nausea he introduced into his scripts were a way of working through the distress he experienced, by allowing him to re-contextualize nausea in a medium over which he had complete control and supervision, with all spontaneity removed from the scenario. His decision to cast women predominantly as the sufferers of nausea then may also point to his tendency to depict his films' women as lacking control over their bodies. In a candid and less politically correct moment in a 1969 interview, he opined, "Women are much less stable than men."[13] In depicting nausea as a predictably female malady, he perhaps assuaged his own fears of losing bodily control.

Apart from employing the baser functions of the body as comedy, or punishment for precious feminine posturing, or for the dramatic effect of existential revulsion, Hitchcock used nausea for rather different purposes in his comedy *Mr. and Mrs. Smith*, and in doing so, revealed an endearing facet of his understanding of love and intimacy. One of the personal stories Hitchcock most enjoyed sharing with friends and colleagues was the telling of the conditions under which he proposed to Alma. In 1924, as he and Alma sailed from Germany to England after having scouted locations for an upcoming feature *The Prude's Fall*, Hitchcock proposed in an unorthodox way.[14]

> The day I proposed to Alma she was lying in an upper bunk of a ship's cabin. The ship was floundering in a most desperate way and so was Alma, who was seasick. I couldn't risk being flowery for fear that in her wretched state she would think I was discussing a movie script. As it was, she groaned, nodded her head and burped. It was one of my greatest scenes—a little weak on dialogue, perhaps, but beautifully staged and not overplayed.

Hitchcock lovingly recounted Alma's belch of assent over the years, and that moment in his life seems to encapsulate their relationship—one built on fondness, familiarity and comfort rather than romance. Hitchcock clearly valued Alma for many reasons, not the least of which was her unconditional acceptance and lack of judgment.

Twice in *Mr. and Mrs. Smith*, Hitchcock employs a reference to the vulgarity of the body only to transform it into a gesture of abiding, if underappreciated, love. First, after Ann Smith (Carole Lombard) has accompanied her husband's business partner Jeff (played by Gene Raymond) on a date, she practically force-feeds him a beaker of brandy (discussed in the following section), and then, when it does not make him sick or misbehaved, she marvels, "What a constitution. . . . The very first time I went out with David, he ruined a brand new $85 dress I had. He was just awful. Didn't change the whole first year we were married." In evoking the comparison between the constitution of the two men, Ann appears to flatter Jeff's masculinity, yet her supposedly exasperated recollection of David's habits of vomiting early in their relationship registers more clearly as a nostalgia for the younger, more reckless days of their marriage, belying the adulation of Jeff.

Later on, as Ann discusses marrying Jeff and taking a boat on their honeymoon, David takes revenge, airing his own reminiscences of Ann's imperfections; he tells her future in-laws: "She's not a very good sailor. Whenever she gets on a boat, don't let her have anything to eat, even if she wants to. Just put her to bed, put a hot-water bottle on her stomach, and hold it there no matter how she hollers. That settles her stomach." While David's intention may have been to embarrass his ex-wife, what comes across much more clearly is his profession of intimacy with and attachment to her, even in moments of discomfort and nausea. The scene almost directly pays tribute to Hitchcock and Alma's engagement. Though intertextual knowledge of his and Alma's betrothal enriches the appreciation of the scene here, it is certainly not necessary to indicate to the audience that husband and wife still regard one another with great fondness and a redemptive knowledge of one another's bodies, even in their abject states, that Hitchcock so cherished in his own life mate.

Hitchcock would often repeat a story that, for him, epitomized the feeling of being deeply in love. He recalls a couple he saw walking in the countryside while on a train from Boulogne to Paris just before the Second World War. "The boy was urinating against a wall and the girl had hold of his arm, never letting go. She would look down at what he was doing, and then look around at the scenery, and down again to see how far he's got on. She couldn't let go. Romance must not be interrupted, even by urinating."[15] Hitchcock often used this anecdote to account for his cinematographic choices in the love scene between Cary Grant and Ingrid Bergman in *Notorious*. In it, the camera trains tightly on the two figures who are intermittently kissing, even as they walk together across the room. The actors reportedly found the scene incredibly awkward in its blocking, though Hitchcock purposefully wanted to convey this sense of unbreakable closeness; he would frequently refer to this taut framing as conveying a spectator's feeling of ménage à trois with Grant and Bergman. His use of this countryside tableau to justify his cinematic rendering of love is another instance in which Hitchcock reveals that love, for him, is strongly dependent on accepting the body of the other unconditionally, in all of its vulgar and vulnerable states.

As my evocation of the above anecdote and the reading of *Mr. and Mrs. Smith* conveys, Hitchcock's deployment of the nauseated woman is not always offered as demeaning spectacle or as a punishing signifier of bodily disenfranchisement. Even in moments of his portraying female bodily alienation through nausea, Hitchcock was possibly identifying with or even empathizing with this disenfranchisement, as much as he evoked the images punitively. Nausea is not just abject spectacle, but a dramatization of the body in revolt. To vomit is to refuse incorporation, to reject that which one has been fed, and to expel it, often as a matter of protection or survival. If we examine *Notorious*'s Alicia in particular, we divine the portrait of a woman who has been fed a steady diet of Nazi propaganda, and then has been force-fed the notion that her most redemptive patriotic function may be to act as a traitorous whore. The nausea that accompanies Alicia's steady consumption of liquor and then poison can be interpreted as Hitchcock's means of demonstrating

Alicia's resistance to the patriarchal narratives that have shaped her into a self-destructive Mata Hari who "makes love for the papers." Alicia's sickness is neither funny, nor does it generate schadenfreude. It stands as a testament to her vulnerability and functions as the last modicum of self-preservation she managed to muster in the face of a deeply misogynist design.

The poetics of potables

It is no secret that Hitchcock had a lifelong, complicated relationship, not just with food, but with drink. By many sets of diagnostic criteria, he would have been considered an alcoholic, though, given his steady and prolific artistic output, he was clearly a high-functioning one. Donald Spoto discusses his habits of alcohol consumption as but one of several facets of the artist's "dark side," and certainly Hitchcock's reliance on alcohol for social lubrication and escapism created problems in his personal and professional life. However, it is not in the purview of this chapter to assess the damages alcohol brought to Hitchcock's relationships or career, but instead to excavate the potentially generative ways that his attitudes toward, and experience with, drinking contributed to his filmmaking.

As Spoto helpfully mentions, of Hitchcock's fifty-three feature films, fifty-one of them contain references to brandy. It was one of Hitchcock's favorite drinks and had a host of connotations that made it a useful part of the mise-en-scene of most of his films. A distilled wine with its production dating back to the Middle Ages, brandy was wrongly thought to have medicinal effects—thus Hitchcock's joyous refrain, "It's not alcohol; it's medicine!"—and is often used in his films to restore someone's vitality after they have fainted or broken down from shock (*Young and Innocent, The Lady Vanishes, Rebecca, North by Northwest, The Birds*, etc.). Brandy is also a customary after-dinner drink, something to be savored in contemplation of the previous meal. In four of Hitchcock's films and episodes of *Alfred Hitchcock Presents*, Hitchcock named supporting characters—two cops, a sailor and a prison inmate—"Hennessey," the most recognizable brand name of cognac in the United States.[16] Given that he often depicted policemen as inept, apathetic, or generally ineffectual, the name Hennessey given to law officers is a nice comic aside (suggesting the idea of agents of the law drinking on the job). The repeated use of the name Hennessey is Hitchcock's intertextual wink at the audience, a confession that he has featured brandy so frequently in his body of work; it has in essence become a character in and of itself.

Brandy contributes to the fate of quite a few characters throughout Hitchcock's work, through its loosening of inhibitions and its slackening of judgment. In *Suspicion*, for instance, the loveable but dimly gullible Beaky is portrayed as vulnerable both to the charms of his friend Johnnie (played by Cary Grant) and to an allergy to brandy, that ultimately costs him his life. Because Lina (played by Joan Fontaine) and the audience have witnessed Johnnie goading Beaky into downing a beaker of brandy early in the film, when news surfaces that Beaky has died from the same gamble while in France, presumably of anaphylactic shock, Johnnie is cast in an even more suspicious light. A brandy decanter becomes a central prop in the murder of Edna Druce in his 1930 *Murder!* When amateur sleuth Sir John Menier (played by Herbert Marshall) discovers a bottle of Martell in Fane the murderer's dressing room, he begins to fill in the missing blanks of the murder scene, where a carafe of brandy has been emptied inexplicably.

The tradition of after-dinner brandy and cigars is portrayed in several Hitchcock films, and in *The Paradine Case* (1947), it takes on greater significance as an indicator of antagonist Lord Horfield's (played by Charles Laughton) perverse preoccupation with maintaining a social order that segregates men from women. After the first dinner scene, Horfield forcefully excuses the women so that the men might partake of brandy and cigars alone. Lady Horfield (Ethel Barrymore) weakly observes that her husband clings to the outmoded tradition, and it becomes clear throughout the film that Horfield entertains misogynist anxieties about the pollution of the public sphere by female sentiment. Frequently, he scolds both wife and daughter for their inquiries about the case over which he is presiding. Repeatedly, he conveys women's inability to make rational, impartial decisions, and he characterizes their inclinations toward mercy and sympathy as illustrative of an inferior intellect. Tellingly, Tony Keane (played by Gregory Peck), who becomes emotionally involved in the fate of his client, declines a cigar that Horfield offers in this segregated masculine space, a refusal to participate in the phallic rites insistently maintained by the judge. Lady Horfield, in the film's final scene, makes her contempt for her husband's impassive nature known, and in damning his regrettable apathy, she breaks her glass of port, which Horfield then throws into the fire. Later, in *Frenzy*, we have a repetition of the breaking of a glass—this time, a brandy snifter—at the dinner table, as Blaney's anger at his wife's financial success in commercializing romance comes to a bitter head.

In addition to brandy, Hitchcock found many cinematic uses for champagne. It was, for him, a beverage of celebration, but also one to be appreciated regularly at lunch and dinner. Around the time he filmed *Foreign Correspondent*, Hitch was known to consume a healthy amount of champagne at lunch, and then would snooze through his afternoon shoot.[17] He titled his 1928 comedy *Champagne*, a light comedy about a girl rebelling against her father, the owner of a prosperous champagne business. Hitchcock used champagne often to convey a celebratory or festive mood through mise-en-scene, and in *Notorious* (1946), he actually used the consumption of champagne to generate suspense. Alicia (Bergman) and Devlin (Grant) explore the wine cellar of her husband Alex (Rains) after having obtained a key to it, and they are only assured safety from detection as long as the champagne supply at the party overhead does not run out. Thus, we have brilliant crosscutting between the leads' discovery of uranium in the wine bottles (the film's famous MacGuffin) and shots of a quickly diminishing number of champagne bottles. Hitchcock takes his cameo in this same scene, as he sips a glass of champagne (and thus, comically contributes to the dangerous discovery of his leads). He later stages a costume party, replete with buckets of champagne, in *To Catch a Thief*, in a similar vein, to provide dramatic contrast between the superficial festivities and the murkier mission of Grant and Kelly, as they attempt to smoke out the true cat burglar.

Although Hitchcock portrayed the consumption of alcohol in all of his films, he rarely thematized dependence on alcohol as a social concern or as a dominant character trait. Robert Benchley's Stebbins in *Foreign Correspondent* (discussed later in the chapter) is an exception, though his alcoholism is not presented as a problem so much as a way of life for which he is nostalgic. Two important exceptions are, of course, Ingrid Bergman's roles in both *Notorious* and *Under Capricorn*. In both roles, Bergman's character drinks out of guilt (derived from, in the first, her father's Nazi activity, and in the second, her husband's banishment). In *Notorious*, Hitchcock couples her heavy drinking with promiscuity, both ineffectual escapes from the sins of her father. In both films, intoxication is explored both as self-medication and as insidious manipulation; both women are drugged or poisoned. *Strangers on a Train* does not explore a character's alcoholism, but it employs a character's intoxication as a plot complication. As Guy desperately searches for an alibi for his wife's murder, he attempts to secure a witness who could place him on a commuter train at the time of her death (at the hands of Guy's foil Bruno). Unfortunately, the passenger who rode with Guy was in the midst of an alcohol-induced blackout. Perhaps more famously, Cary Grant's Roger Thornhill of *North by Northwest* is force-fed a large quantity of alcohol so that his fatal car crash could be construed as the product of drunk driving.

The coerced consumption of dangerous amounts of liquor in *North by Northwest* is an extreme and exaggerated variation on a dramatic situation quite common in the Hitchcock oeuvre. His films are rife with examples of characters' wielding power over another or revealing their more cloaked desires in their asking or gently forcing characters to consume what they desire them to. In some instances, it is a loving gesture, an indication of concern or tough love. In others, it is a selfish calculation intended to disarm the consumer. In still others, it is a gesture of malice. Hitchcock recognized the dramatic potential inherent in the simple act of sharing a drink and mined it for the dramatic elements that drinking together could conjure. Issues of trust, companionship, willpower, manipulation, loyalty, and compliance are all condensed in the host/guest scenario, and Hitchcock understood that a small gesture could read quite large on the film screen.

Spoto calls Hitchcock's "most personal" touch in his romantic comedy *Mr. and Mrs. Smith* the moment in which Carole Lombard's forcefully instructs to Gene Raymond to drink: "This isn't alcohol—it's medicine. It kills the germs. All in one gulp!" He goes on to report (somewhat inaccurately) that in the following years, there are a dozen instances of dialogue that is punctuated with the classic validating excuse that Hitchcock's off-screen companions heard so often: "It isn't alcohol; it's like medicine!" The purpose of Spoto's observation seems to be to illustrate the frequency with which Hitchcock would deflect or diffuse observations about his own drinking with humor, and how he would similarly characterize drinkers in his films as making such excuses. In reality, there are only four such instances that characterize alcohol as medicinal or remedial in some form. As the chart below reveals, however, there are many more instances of characters offering inducements to drink. These moments of exhortation can function as moments of suspense or revelation. In the cases of *The Lady Vanishes* and *Notorious* (and, including non-verbal inducement, *Suspicion*), the offer of a drink bears dramatic weight because the drinks offered are drugged or poisoned. In *Rebecca*, *Stage Fright*, and *Vertigo*, the men's persuasion to drink indicates a benign, if slightly condescending, paternalism, and the women's obedience demonstrate trust. In *North by Northwest*, enticement to drink is a sardonically intended toast, expressing Thornhill's distrust of Eve Kendall (Eva Marie Saint).

The exhortation to "Drink it down," "Finish it," or "All in one gulp" discloses more about Hitchcock's relation to consumption than his use of these scenarios to explicate power relations between characters. They also point to his own idiosyncratic habits of consumption. In his *Dark Side of Genius*, Spoto reports on Hitchcock's dining habits in the mid to late 1950s: "Before lunch at Santa Cruz, he liked to drink a tumblerful of Cointreau . . . consumed in one great swallow, after a furtive glance to see that Alma was out of sight."[18] Supportive of him in every other aspect of his life, Alma was concerned by, and vigilant over, Hitchcock's consumption of food and drink. His habits of gulping food and beverage may have been initiated as a means of eluding Alma's policing, but he clearly internalized this surveillance, and ingested quickly regardless of whether or not Alma was present. According to Herbert Coleman, Hitchcock's longtime assistant director, "He always said he hated the idea of swallowing food and drink, and in fact everything seemed to be taken in one huge gulp." Spoto characterizes this tendency as one of the "odd habits of a man who perhaps loved the idea of being sated more than the act of ingestion, which somehow seemed to him indelicate and reminded him of nausea and sexual activity—connections he frequently made to dining companions at inappropriate moments."[19]

It may seem incongruous that a man of carefully cultivated tastes, who spent a great deal of time and money planning meals, describing them, preparing them, and recalling them fondly, should be loathe to savor the process of eating and drinking. Hitchcock accounted for this disconnect as he addressed the New York press after finishing his legendary three-steak meal at the 21 Club: "I find contentment from food. It is a mental process rather than a physical one." His carefully chosen words strikingly echo his often repeated contention that, in the act of filmmaking, he received great pleasure from conceiving the story and building the film frame by frame in his mind, but was in fact rather bored by the time of the shooting, which entailed the physical translation of the ideal film in his head into the final product, which never quite measured up. Because food was the stuff of his fantasy, its actual ingestion perhaps paled in comparison to his contemplation of it.

The disparity between the ideal and the real may explain part of Hitchcock's habits of quick ingestion. Yet I am compelled by another possibility that speaks to the major concerns of this study. Because Hitchcock was almost compulsively concerned with having control over himself and his surroundings, the one arena in which he was ineffectual at establishing control—his consumption of food and drink—had to have constituted a source of deep shame. Hitchcock joked frequently about his weight, rarely broaching the subject of fat shame in his daily life, though on occasion he would articulate these feelings with great pathos. In one instance, he confided to Charlotte Chandler,

> When I look into my mirror, I don't see Cary Grant. I look into my mirror as little as possible, because the person who looks back at me has always seemed something of a stranger who doesn't look at all the way I feel. But, somehow, he kept getting into my mirror.[20]

Even as he attempts to inject this confession with the same levity he employed in his comedic speeches "The Real Me (The Thin One)," which I have discussed at length in Chapter 2, the anguish he feels about his weight is palpable. The "stranger" in the mirror constitutes an almost violent disavowal of his actual material body, a will-to-disembodiment, perhaps. From this confession, we learn that Hitchcock's fatness endowed him with a nightmarish sense of the inescapable uncanny, a tragically irreconcilable estrangement from his own self-image. For these reasons, I contend, the act of ingestion and, more importantly *being watched* in the act of ingestion, was incredibly fraught for Hitchcock. As much as he loved food and drink, and enjoyed company at the dinner table, the physical, mechanical act of ingestion made him feel naked, vulnerable, and ashamed. Ingestion constituted proof that, through his lack of self-control in this one aspect of his life, he was contributing to the traitorous body that he so anxiously disavowed in self-contemplation. The fact that he would liken the process of eating and drinking to that of vomiting and having sex foregrounds this mental connection he automatically forged between acts that would render the body vulnerable, captured in the throes of a pleasure that signified his own loss of control.

"Drink It Down": An Hitchcockian imperative

The Lady Vanishes (1937)	Dr. Hartz (Paul Lukas) to Iris (Margaret Lockwood), hoping to poison her.	"Drink. That will settle your nerves. To your health. Come on! Drink!"
Rebecca (1940)	Maxim (Laurence Olivier) to the Second Mrs. De Winter (Joan Fontaine), loving, but condescending order.	"Finish your eggs like a good girl." And later, handing her brandy, "It'll do you good."
Mr. and Mrs. Smith (1941)	Ann Smith (Carole Lombard) to Jeff (Gene Raymond), trying to get him drunk on a date, in hopes that he will be responsive to her.	"Two big swallows of this, and there'll be one less pneumonia case tomorrow. All in one big gulp. This isn't alcohol, Jeff, it's medicine. One big gulp now. It's just medicine; it kills the germs. All in one gulp now."
Spellbound (1945)	Dr. Alex Brulov (Michael Chekhov) to John Ballantyne (Gregory Peck), trying to drug him unconscious, in self-defense.	"Nobody likes to have milk by himself. We will drink to you, to when we are young and know nothing but living."
Notorious (1946)	T. R. Devlin (Cary Grant) to Alicia Huberman (Ingrid Bergman), trying to cure her hangover.	"You'd better drink that. Go on, drink it. Finish it. You'll feel better."

(Continued)

Notorious (1946)	Alex Sebastian (Claude Rains) to Alicia (Bergman), trying to slowly poison her.	"Drink your coffee, darling, it's getting cold."
Stage Fright (1950)	Ordinary Smith (Michael Wilding) to Eve Gill (Jane Wyman), trying to revive her after she feels faint.	"This little brandy can't do you any harm. Why not drink it?"
Stage Fright (1950)	Jonathan (Richard Todd) to Charlotte Inwood (Marlene Dietrich) in his fabricated account of the murder.	"I thought I had brandy. . . . Here, drink this!"
The Man Who Knew Too Much (1956)	Ben McKenna (Jimmy Stewart) to Jo McKenna (Doris Day), trying to sedate her before she learns of her son's kidnapping.	"I want you to take these; they'll relax you. I'm the doctor, Jo, you know what happens when you get excited. I know you'll feel better if you take these. Don't fight me on this one."
North By Northwest (1959)	Roger Thornhill (Cary Grant) to Eve (Eva Marie Saint), toasting them (disingenuously) with scotch.	"To us. A long and lasting friendship."
North By Northwest (1959)	Van Damm (James Mason) to Eve (Saint) and Leonard (Martin Landau), toasting with champagne, before he plans to kill her.	"To you, my dear, and all the lovely moments that we've had together. Jump in, Leonard, the champagne's fine."
Vertigo (1958)	Scottie (Jimmy Stewart) to Judy (Kim Novak), plying her with brandy as she is breaking down.	"Here, Judy, drink this straight down, just like medicine."
Topaz (1969)	Jacques Granville (Michel Piccoli) to Henri Jarre (Philippe Noiret), trying to get him out of his apartment in order to make a rendezvous.	"This will settle your nerves. Now, if you will finish that cognac."

Lactose and intolerance: The poisonous meanings of milk

If Hitchcock used liquor in the service of staging festivity, confrontation, social manipulation, and escapism, and signifying pleasure, he used milk to signify, in many ways, alcohol's antithesis. From Hitch's earliest days in Hollywood, milk was already a staple of the middle-class home and a signifier of hygienic, healthy living. By the 1940s the National Dairy Council had launched an aggressive ad campaign for milk, proselytizing America's heartland with its many promises: "Good teeth. Vitality. Endurance. Strong bones."[21] Then, as now, milk came to stand for the wholesome positive values of the bourgeoisie—a thoroughly suburban beverage, and its strong connotative powers did not escape Hitchcock. Milk first appears in an American Hitchcock film in *Foreign Correspondent* (1941) as protagonist Johnny Jones (played by Joel McCrea) arrives in London on assignment to report on subversive activity of the Axis Powers. His contact Stebbins (played by Robert Benchley), upon meeting Johnny, orders them "a scotch and soda, and a glass of milk." When Johnny inquires about the milk, Stebbins explains that he has been ordered "on the wagon" by his doctor, who warned him that unless he abstained for a month, he could look for a new set of organs. Stebbins watches Johnny drink the scotch and soda longingly, hoping for vicarious pleasure by asking how it tastes. "Just like any scotch and soda," Johnny responds, to which Stebbins replies, pining, "I thought so." Then, upon taking a sip of his milk, he complains, "Doesn't taste the same as when I was a baby; tastes like poison."[22]

Correspondent's Stebbins is a figure of comic relief in an often white-knuckle film shot through with hot pursuits, double-crossings, and adrenaline-laced set pieces. Stebbins is the avuncular lush—who seems not to have let anything as wholesome as milk pass his lips since infancy—who provides an emotional anchor to the unknown land of Jones's assignment. The notion that milk—in comparison with the hard liquor he craves—"tastes like poison" establishes him as hopelessly vice-ridden, but also endearing to the audience—a commonly coupled set of attributes for Hitchcock's characters. Sadly, life imitated art in this instance; Benchley died of complications from cirrhosis of the liver at fifty-six, just five years later. The comic reversal of expectation, whereby milk is experienced as toxic, and liquor, as bestowing vitality, is simultaneously a nod to the life of pleasure championed by Hitchcock and a gesture of disdain for the bland conformity and numbing wholesomeness of the nuclear family that keeps milk circulating.

In the year following *Foreign Correspondent*, a glass of milk is the focus in one of Hitchcock's most memorable set pieces of the early 1940s. The iconic "glowing milk" of his 1941 *Suspicion*, starring Joan Fontaine and Cary Grant, stands at center of one of the penultimate scenes of the film. Grant's Johnnie prepares a bedtime glass of warm milk ostensibly to calm the nerves of his wife Lina, who has been driven nearly to distraction by the growing belief that Johnnie intends to kill her in order to collect on her life insurance policy. As Grant famously carries the glass of milk up the dark staircase, the milk glows ominously—clearly a visual declaration of Hitchcock's German Expressionist roots a la Murnau—as the audience wonders if the milk is, in fact, poisoned. Hitchcock had placed a light bulb in the milk glass, so that it would be even more pronounced against the dark staircase and Grant's dark robe. In the original script, Grant is actually a killer; Lina drinks the milk, knowing it is poisoned, a tragically romantic gesture proclaiming her refusal to live in a world without Johnnie's love. Yet she has also written a letter incriminating Johnnie before she drinks the lethal milk, and Johnnie, after ensuring that she is dead, whistles while carrying the sealed letter out to the mailbox, unaware that he is contributing to his own capture.

Because both the Production Code and consultation with producers at RKO revealed that Grant could never get away with playing a cold-blooded killer, the ending was modified. Grant turns out to be little more than an irresponsible cad, and Lina has imagined his murderous tendencies. The milk scene dissolves to the following morning, with a close-up on the untouched milk glass and Lina preparing a suitcase to leave Johnnie for her mother's house. In two films a year apart, we have a joke about milk's poisonous taste and milk that may or not be laced with poison. The idea of poisoned milk seems all the more insidious because it *is* so wholesome and cozy, something one (often a child) drinks at bedtime as a soporific.

A drugged milk concoction plays a role in 1945's *Spellbound* several years later. In the scene in question, amnesiac John Ballantyne (played by Gregory Peck) has been triggered by the color white with lines in it (a symbol that connects with his submerged memory of a murder on the ski slopes), and in a sort of semiconscious hypnotic state, he wields a razor, nearing the sleeping Constance (played by Ingrid Bergman), before deciding better of it and descending the stairs, where he meets the still-awake mentor of Constance, Dr. Alex Brulov. Brulov realizes right away that that the psychosis has consumed Ballantyne and offers him a glass of milk that he has spiked with bromide. In a fascinating POV shot, the camera is placed in the perspective of Ballantyne as he quickly drains the glass of milk while watching Brulov across the room. The POV then fades to white (appropriate because of the milk he has just downed and the snow, which is his visual amnesiac trigger), indicating that Ballantyne has lost consciousness, and the scene segues into the next morning, where Constance wakes to find John missing from the bedroom, and hears from Alex that he had to subdue her murderous lover with the drugged milk. Again, we have the dissonant (though felicitous) combination of wholesome soporific and dangerous toxin—a pairing that clearly gave Hitchcock some degree of pleasure in its dramatic reiteration in different contexts. Michael Walker, in his book *Hitchcock's Motifs*, smartly complicates the scenario by suggesting that bromide, used in the Second World War to decrease sexual potency, heightens the portrayal of the sexually charged Oedipal triangle formed by Constance, John, and her mentor/father figure Brulov. Thus, besides containing the threat that John in his psychosis poses, Brulov lessens the sexual threat that the younger, more virile John has implicitly issued in his romantic claims to Constance.[23]

Milk makes a brief appearance in 1955's *To Catch a Thief*, when a chef, contemptuous of John Robie (Cary Grant), pours milk into a saucer and offers it to him, implying that he knows that Robie is The Cat, responsible for a recent slew of thefts. The last time milk makes a particularly meaningful appearance in a Hitchcock film occurs about ten years after *Spellbound*, in the 1955 film *The Trouble With Harry*, one of his more darkly humorous suspense films. The film takes place in a small wholesome community of Vermont, and slowly the simple, placid, down-home exterior of the town is stripped away to reveal the rather morbid, sometimes scandalous secrets of its inhabitants. The plot revolves around the repeated discovery of the corpse of a man named Harry. The physical comedy of the film derives from the many characters' manipulation of the corpse—where they put him, the stories they tell about him—and the story reveals that the wholesome and innocent Jennifer (played by Shirley MacLaine, in her first cinematic role) believes she has murdered Harry by braining him with a milk bottle.

In three of the four situations involving the drinking (or almost drinking) of milk, the character drinking the milk is either emasculated or effeminized. Stebbins of *Foreign Correspondent* has been forced to abstain from one of his few pleasures in life and a crutch for dealing with its adversities; the submissive and terrorized Lina contemplates murder at the hand of her husband, given over to fatalistic feelings of powerlessness; and the feminized patient John Ballantyne—at the mercy of his lost memory and vulnerable because of his fugitive status—is administered the drug by Doctor Brulov.

Yet, in the fourth scenario, milk as a pivotal prop undergoes a transformation in terms of its signifying power. Jennifer, the wife who has opted to leave her husband and start over on her own terms, wields the milk bottle as a symbol of power against him. The object of banal domesticity is used to preserve her independence and sovereignty in the home. In a film that trades heavily in sex-and-food jokes—some of which will be explored later—this unexpected reversal has resonance in its depiction of power's fluidity. Milk appears in other

Hitchcock films, though mostly in the background. *Psycho*'s Marion Crane, for example, is served milk and sandwiches by Norman Bates in the scene preceding her murder—another ironic instance of the cozy domestic gone awry.[24] In *Rear Window*, L. B. Jefferies lunches on milk and sandwiches in his wheelchair, prepared by his nurse Stella. From the above examples, it follows that milk is usually consumed by a character in a vulnerable or dependent position, much like the infant who nurses.

A year or so after the release of *Psycho* (1960), a man was apprehended for murdering three women in Los Angeles, and in a statement to the press, he revealed that he had watched *Psycho* before committing his third murder. Anxious to get a scoop on the impact of movie violence on social behavior, reporters went directly to Hitchcock to get his official comment. Hitchcock, disgusted with the simplistic reasoning of the "hypodermic needle theory" of media's social influence on human behavior, retorted, "I'd like to know what film he watched before he committed the second murder. And perhaps before the first murder, he drank a glass of milk!" Clearly the rhetorical thrust of Hitchcock's response was an evocation of the *post hoc* fallacy involved in assigning causality to the relationship between movie violence and real crime, but in light of Hitchcock's past dramatizations of milk in violent and dangerous contexts, his allusion, as usual, has an element of the tongue in cheek as well.

Hitchcockian consumption and the carnivalesque

The variously lusty, depraved, hearty, and surprising appetites that Hitchcock's characters display should signal to us that acts of consumption in the world of his films carry strong interpretive weight. Mikhail Bakhtin's concept of the carnivalesque, as theorized in *Rabelais and His World*, is energizing to this study in its potential to illuminate aspects of Hitchcock's various textual worlds, concerned as they are with excessive and idiosyncratic consumption. Characterized by the inversion of social and political hierarchy and a celebration of the low stratum—the bodily, particularly, the womb, stomach, anus, penis—over the upper—the soul, the intellect, the carnivalesque as a cultural mode creates a terrain that casts as the center those typically marginalized by social hierarchies. Bakhtin describes the carnival as a space that simultaneously emphasizes collectivity and destabilizes conventional categories of identity that typically constitute social hierarchy. "All were considered equal during carnival. Here, in the town square, a special form of free and familiar contact reigned among people who were usually divided by the barriers of caste, property, profession, and age."[25] Hitchcock's films by and large do not participate in the construction of a wholly carnivalesque universe; they rely too much on existing hierarchies for their dramatic thrust, even when they tweak or question those hierarchies. Yet carnival as a mode of sensory and social experience forms part of the fabric of many of his films. To begin with, five of his films—*Murder!* (1930), *Mr. and Mrs. Smith* (1941), *Saboteur* (1942), *Stage Fright* (1950), and *Strangers on a Train* (1951)—contain literal scenes of carnival that stage, if not total social inversion, then at least a subversive re-imagining of characters and their place in the world. For Hitchcock, as for Bakhtin, the carnival is a site of excessive consumption and perverse performance, often bordering on the grotesque, and allows for the emergence of voices and unconventional pleasures that have been muted in other registers of the picture.

The depiction of carnival is somewhat marginal in Hitchcock's early film *Murder!*, though, like *Strangers on a Train*, its climax stages the demise of its villain within the space of the carnival (in this case, a circus). The cast is composed mostly of members of a theatrical company, and the film depicts a murder within the community of the theater. The actual murderer, however, is a member of the acting troupe, but also an acrobat in the circus. While the theatrical group is portrayed as living on society's margins socioeconomically, the circus is figured as yet more marginal. The secret that murderer Fane carries—that he is "half-caste"—concerns his social illegitimacy, and the carnival signifies as that space that houses, if not embraces, the abject seeking asylum. The fact that Fane cross-dresses in his trapeze act and in his theatrical roles simultaneously renders him more exotic and abject, yet at home in the carnival's pageantry. It is through the mode of the carnivalesque that Hitchcock establishes a dramatic tension between the pathos evoked by Fane's racial abjection and the sensational perversity of his murderous sexual deviance.

Saboteur takes an interesting detour through the carnivalesque as fugitive protagonist Barry Kane (Robert Cummings) and love interest Pat (Priscilla Lane), having been stranded in the Nevada desert, find refuge and sanctuary from the police in a circus caravan containing its sideshow performers. The "human oddities" of the Russell Brothers Circus take the couple under their wing, protecting them from officers searching each car for Kane, an archetypal Hitchcockian "wrong man" who has been blamed for the sabotage of an airbase. The motley crew consists of Bones, the human skeleton; the Major, a fascist dwarf styled like Hitler; "Siamese" twins Minnie and Marigold; Fat Lady Titania; and Bearded Lady Esmerelda. Though some are hesitant to embrace the fleeing couple, they collectively decide to aid their fellow travelers with no questions asked. Hitchcock developed this respite from the film's cross-country chase in order to vary the pace and to provide a locus of comedy and poignancy that had to that point been missing from the film. The circus performers, who have clearly been marginalized by their exceptional bodies, have come to expect coldhearted treatment from the "normals," and recognize the importance of compassion, and in an ironic reversal of expectation, these "oddities" turn out to have the most humane intentions and the greatest sense of compassion of all that the couple encounters throughout the film.

Strangers on a Train is perhaps the most interesting engagement of the Bakhtinian carnival in all of Hitchcock's work, particularly as the characters Miriam and Bruno evoke the perversity of the grotesque, through their marginal sexual identities and the free rein given their libidos in the space of the carnival. Bakhtin argues that the figure that most effectively condenses the excessive, grotesque qualities of the carnivalesque is that of the pregnant hag—a figure that is old yet somehow still fertile, sexually licentious, and laughing. Miriam, protagonist Guy's current wife, who is presented dramatically as one of the two major obstacles to Guy's assumption of legitimate heterosexual relations (Bruno being the other), is a fascinatingly carnivalesque character. She is indeed pregnant and promiscuous enough to obscure paternal knowledge with any certainty.[26] Bruno stalks Miriam, following her to the fair, where she brings not one but two dates with her. Once at the fair, she is not only voracious in terms of food, but also sexually insatiable. Despite the fawning of her two beaux, she becomes aroused by Bruno's attentions and encourages his close pursuit. As they stand in line for ice cream cones, Miriam complains, "I should have had a hot dog first. It would have satisfied my craving a little better." Her two dates joke back, "Craving for what?" "I don't know where you put it all," and "I never saw a girl eat so much in all my life." Clearly, the question "Craving for what?" has a sexual connotation, indicating a confusion or conflation of sexual appetites with hunger for food, and the phallic aspect of the hot dog is invoked in his teasing. "I don't know where you put it all" references the disparity between Miriam's insatiable appetite and her thin physique—the exact opposite of the disparity that the large yet reportedly moderate Hitchcock faced in his daily life.

The idea of Miriam's thinness despite her great appetites suggests either a parasitism, the notion that something is feeding on her (and, of course, this is literally true because of her pregnancy) or a sense of abnormal satiety—that she cannot be satisfied sexually or otherwise by normal diet. Besides consuming food—she eats ice cream, asks for hot dogs and then popcorn, which one of her beaux nixes, saying, "It's no fun necking with a mouthful of popcorn"—she leads her dates through a labyrinth of archetypal carnival spaces: the Strong Man game, the coin tosses, the carousel, the Tunnel of Love, ensuring at each stop that Bruno is still pursuing her. The film connects the perversely antagonizing Miriam not just with excessive consumption, but also with waste and abjection. When Guy announces his intention to divorce her and marry

Anne Morton, Miriam defiantly responds, "You can throw all your little thoughts of her right into the ashcan!" and, later, "You can't throw me away like an old shoe!" At the scene of her death, we witness Bruno choking her, throttling her at the very site of consumption and ingestion, as the image is refracted to us through the funhouse mirrorlike distortions of her broken spectacles.[27]

Realized by Hitchcock ten years prior to *Strangers on a Train*, the titular character of *Rebecca*, though bodily absent from the film, operates through a similar semiotic to that of the Bakhtinian hag that typifies the carnivalesque. Though Hitchcock does not stage a proper scene of carnival in *Rebecca*, he does portray the costume ball, a scene that Rebecca dominates and ruins (with the aid of Mrs. Danvers), even in her absence. In the vein of the carnival and its grotesque consumption, the villainous Rebecca prefigures *Strangers* villain Miriam in intriguing ways. Like Miriam, Rebecca uses the notion of pregnancy to enrage and barter with the lead male. Both women threaten to bring forth a monstrous child as a means of consigning their lovers to a life of abjection and stigma—Rebecca, by providing Manderley a bastard heir outside the de Winter bloodline, and Miriam, by making it impossible for Guy to abandon her in favor of the upwardly mobile Morton dynasty. Like Miriam, Rebecca is revealed to be sexually voracious and conniving. Rebecca's characterization as grotesque, in fact, surpasses that of Miriam; she is portrayed as incestuous, having an affair with her cousin, the effete Jack Favell, and she also uses the occasion of her pending cancerous death to stage a fake pregnancy, thereby unleashing a host of perverse connections between fetal growth and malignant cancerous growth from within. She ends, of course, where the monstrous feminine must end up—on the ocean floor, devoured by the maternal grave of the sea.

Finally, just as *Strangers*'s Miriam is linked to trash and abjection through her dialogue (the "ash can," the "old shoe"), Rebecca is similarly yoked to the semiotics of refuse and excess. As Maxim makes his confession in the boathouse, an ashtray overflowing with cigarette butts stands in for the absent Rebecca. The image of this filthy overflow is meaningful to Hitchcock, particularly as he copped several times to an obsessive-compulsive need to be the "ashtray-emptier" in any social situation. He intends, then, for this object-surrogate for Rebecca's presence to be a disturbing one. The other objects that stand in for the absent Rebecca are either those of bodily intimacy or ones that bespeak an egomaniacal excess: along with "I," the audience is introduced to Rebecca by the devoted Mrs. Danvers through the intimacy of her lingerie, prepared "by the nuns of St. Clair," and her presence is also made palpable through the excessive piles of monogrammed stationery, pillowcases, and linen. Tellingly, when the second Mrs. De Winter finally comes into her own as lady of the house, her first instruction is to have the monogrammed office accouterments destroyed. And of course, the film's final image is that of the burning monogrammed pillow case. Thus, in both *Rebecca* and *Strangers on a Train*, Hitchcock employs the concept of the wayward female appetite to evince a perverse villainy that is paradoxically both potent and abject.

Yet, Hitchcock does not limit his characterizations of the perverse and voracious consumer to his female characters. In the figure of his antagonist Bruno Anthony in *Strangers on a Train*, he couples questionable consumption with perverse sexuality. Bruno, the other figure of excess and perversity in the film, also seems to thrive in the carnival atmosphere. He bursts the balloon of a child who has attempted to ambush him with a toy gun, and in so doing, demonstrates a callous lack of sentimentality, reminiscent of Hitchcock himself. He pursues Miriam with a chilling intensity and single-mindedness of purpose. He may be considered weak and "soft" in the outside world—he repeatedly expresses admiration for men who "do something," he has a clear homoerotic attraction to Guy, and he lives a dandy's life of decadent leisure—but in the space of the carnival, he becomes powerful and masculine. As Miriam's two beaux prove too weak to win her a prize in the sledgehammer game, Bruno steps up and not only rings the bell, but off screen, we hear an amazed, "I think he broke it!" from the gathering crowd. This display of strong virility anticipates the murder of Miriam soon to come, where he drains the life from her with his bare hands. Bruno's hypermasculine performance suggests that the carnival is indeed a site of power's inversion, where the effete dandy is transmogrified into a formidable he-man.

In this assessment of Hitchcockian carnival and consumption, it is important to consider the fact that, though both Miriam and Bruno's hungers are given form and voice in the space of the carnival, it is here that they both meet their deaths—Miriam, at the hands of Bruno, and Bruno, as a casualty of the carousel that has careened out of control. Sabrina Barton, in her wonderful essay, "Criss-Cross: Paranoia and Projection in *Strangers on a Train*," describes the carousel's dismantling as a vertiginous display of the mechanisms of normative and coercive heterosexuality collapsing on themselves, both representing chaos, but also a re-ordering whereupon the queer Bruno is exorcized from the film so that Guy can safely re-couple with Anne and escape the challenge to his identity that Bruno's presence elicited. The death of these two subversive characters in the carnival scenario indicates that a Bakhtinian social and sexual inversion is by no means complete, final, or without consequences. The feminine and the queer grotesque perform brilliantly and subversively, but are ultimately contained in the very environment in which their perversity could be articulated.

The carnival scene of *Mr. and Mrs. Smith* (1941) is quite brief, and does not house the same sort of perversities that *Strangers* does with such abandon, but still constitutes a site of transgression. It is to the fair that Ann Smith takes her date Jeff, her husband's business partner and supposedly his best friend. Although, according to the contrived plot, Ann is not technically married to David as she had believed for several years, her dalliance and attempted seduction of Jeff still reads as transgressive behavior, particularly because by the end of the film, true to the structure of the Cavellian remarriage comedy, the couple is reunited with a new conviction about their love. In this carnival scene, Ann takes Jeff up in a parachute ride, and they become comically caught at the top, when it begins to rain heavily on them. Ann's attempt at seduction is thwarted, resulting in Jeff's catching a cold, and the second part of her plan—to get Jeff intoxicated, backfires as well, as he moves from awkwardly frigid to nearly catatonic, with no display of the inhibitions she had hoped to tap. Thus, the sexual appetite and license evoked by the carnivalesque is comically foreclosed for Ann despite her best efforts to the contrary.

The carnivalesque garden party in *Stage Fright* (1950) is rather more multivalent and is employed for several dramatic purposes. Hitchcock was not happy with the film overall, though in his interviews with Truffaut, he expressed a well-justified fondness for its garden party scenes. It is a site of both riveting dramatic tension and wonderful comic relief. The fairground of the party is also a decidedly feminine space, as women play a pivotal part in the several important transactions of the carnival. Conspicuous consumption is played up in the carnival scenes, particularly through the character Chubby Bannister (played by Pat Hitchcock), who shows great fondness for both men and ice cream. Nellie Goode, the greedy blackmailer (who has already shown an inappropriate hunger for money, attention and gin and lemon at her local pub), makes her successful play for hush money at the fairgrounds, extracting money from Eve's father in exchange for her silence about the whereabouts of fugitive Jonathan. Rather comically, as part of a contrivance to force Charlotte Inwood to show her guilt in the murder of her husband, Eve's father tries to win a doll playing a duck-shooting game, hosted by the delightfully toothy character actress Joyce Grenfell (remembered for her hilarious barking, "Lovely Ducks! Lovely Ducks!"). The Commodore's unsuccessful attempts at cheating in order to win the doll provide comedy and generate suspense regarding the completion of their plan to secure Charlotte's guilt.

Commodore Gill finally procures the doll, whereupon they bloody the front of its dress (using the Commodore's actual blood—another nod to the fluids of the carnivalesque) to taunt Charlotte for her blood-soiled dress at the murder scene. Eve and her father then enlist a child—a boy scout—to carry the doll to Charlotte as she performs onstage. The image of the approaching child is disarming, as the doll appears streaked with menstrual blood, producing the same perverse sexual illogic that governs the figure of the Bakhtinian pregnant hag. However, instead of a figure of postmenopausal fertility, we have one of premenstrual ripeness. The presentation of the bloodied doll works to unsettle Charlotte, who has wrongly assumed the doll is a gift from an admiring fan, and thus her crime (for which she is partially responsible, though not culpable as Eve has come to believe) comes to the foreground. The carnival displays the impressive agency of two of the film's women—Eve's aggressive detection and Nellie's successful financial extortion—but it also evokes women's duplicity, avarice, and guilty consumption. This, Hitchcock's use of the carnivalesque, is far from penetrating social criticism, but it certainly demonstrates Hitchcock's fascination and at least partial affinity with the social margins, especially when that marginality is linked with transgressive consumption.

Food, sex, murder: The Hitchcockian trinity of pleasure

One of the reasons Hitchcock's films are so universally appealing is that they thrive on a synergy that comes from mutually reinforcing iconographies of pleasure. We are never simply fed by one stream of visual or narrative pleasure, but rather by a network of connotations, metaphors, allusions, and associations. The semiotics of food, sex, and murder are steeped in one another's imaginative reserves, and they flourish for the spectator in their rhythmically intertwining chains of signification. At his best, Hitchcock braids the vicariously experienced pleasures of consumption, coition, and aestheticized aggression so that the audience can feel these pleasures only in concert, in their rich combinations.

Empirically speaking, given Hitchcock's encyclopedic culinary and criminal knowledge and his quite rudimentary sexual knowledge, it makes sense that Hitchcock depicted pleasures derived from food, sex, and murder in concert. In the mise-en-scenes of desire that permeate his filmmaking, food appears at moments in metonymic relation to sex and violence, and at other moments in a metaphoric capacity. Framed otherwise, the pleasures of food either substitute for or exist alongside sexual fulfillment and the catharsis of unleashed aggression. In a conversation with Charlotte Chandler, Hitchcock mused, "I believe that there is a perfect relationship between love of food and a healthy libido. People who like to eat have a stronger libido, a greater interest in sex." In this profession, Hitchcock was of course revealing something about himself, his twinned preoccupations with food and sex, but he was also pointing out their coextensive signifying powers. A staggering number of his aphorisms about filmmaking rest on the metaphoric and metonymic associations among food, sex, and murder. Consider a few:

- Revenge is sweet and not fattening.
- Man does not live by murder alone. He needs affection, approval, encouragement, and occasionally, a hearty meal.
- Film your murders like love scenes, and your love scenes like murders.[28]
- I do not believe in raw sex. I like my sex cooked, preferably with a delicate sauce.
- A murder without gleaming scissors is like asparagus without the hollandaise sauce—tasteless.

Addressing this primal linkage of themes, David Sterritt calls his later work *Frenzy* "no easy case of a hungry man packing his movie full of eats . . . a complex work charged with oral anxieties and a revealing tendency to couple food imagery with those favorite Hitchcock concerns: sex, violence, and death. (The same linkage can be traced through . . . *Blackmail*, *Suspicion*, *Notorious*, *Rope*, and *Psycho*, among others)."[29] Indeed, these hybrid thematics run throughout the Hitchcock oeuvre.

The consumption of food at times signifies the sublimation of sexual desires in Hitchcock's films, but more often, culinary pleasures are contiguous to, rather than substitutive for, sexual pleasures. One of the most transparent depictions of food as sublimation lies in the opening shots of *Mr. and Mrs. Smith*. Before we ever meet the protagonists, the camera pans slowly over a veritable landscape of dirty dinner dishes, piled across the bedroom floor. Through the servants' exposition, we learn that Ann and David have been fighting for eight days, and that they never leave their bedroom until a quarrel has been resolved. The comically exaggerated display of dirty dishes (over 50) suggests more than the regular accumulation of food over the course of eight days; it suggests that, in lieu of lovemaking, the couple has been preoccupied with eating, channeling their passion into their stomachs. In *The Trouble with Harry*, the awkward and sexually timid Captain Wiles (Edmund Gwenn) and Miss Gravely (Mildred Natwick) disclose their romantic feelings for one another predominantly through a discussion of blueberry muffins.

Food often figures into romantic courtship or sexual foreplay in Hitchcock's universe. Sam Marlowe (John Forsythe) of *The Trouble with Harry* pledges to provide his intended (Shirley MacLaine) with strawberries (her "favorite thing in the world"), "two boxes a month, in and out of season, forever." As John and

Constance are alone for the first time in *Spellbound*, John offers her a choice of sandwich, and her gushing reply, "Liverwurst," indicates her acceptance of the food as a deeply romantic gesture. When asked later by a colleague about the mustard stain on her shirt, she again lovingly replies, "Liverwurst." Eve Kendall (Eva Marie-Saint) in *North by Northwest* makes herself sexually available to Thornhill (Grant) almost immediately, but first recommends the brook trout for dinner, which she describes as "A little trouty but quite good." In a brazenly explicit linkage of culinary pleasures with sexual ones, she informs her paramour, "I never discuss love on an empty stomach."[30]

Grace Kelly's Lisa Freemont of *Rear Window* makes her sexual and romantic intentions with Jeffries (Stewart) known from her introduction, when she brings him the beautiful lobster and frites dinner from the 21 Club. Filmmaker Peter Bogdanovich comments on the idealized portrayal of Lisa by Kelly, and suggests that the meal she brings as proof of her affection is similarly ideal, almost untouchable. The problem with the meal is, in effect, the problem Jeffries has with Lisa. He claims with dismay, "Lisa, it's perfect." The protagonist of *Rebecca* is portrayed as initially wispy, timid, and girlish, and her eating habits—skipping meals, picking at scrambled eggs—reflect this constitution. Throughout the film, particularly after Rebecca's boat is found, "I" truly comes into her own, dramatically assuming an air of strength, confidence, and sexual maturity that eluded her as a new bride. This remarkable growth finds its reinforcement in her attitude toward food; by the end, she displays an appetite, and brings a hearty picnic to fortify Maxim and her during the taxing inquisition regarding Rebecca's death. The girl who could barely pick at a few eggs now produces an abundant basket, laden with chicken, loaves of bread, and champagne.

Hitchcock scholarship has traditionally characterized the auteur as profoundly male-identified, both in his everyday life, and in his cinematic attachments to character. The notion of his desire for the female cinematic object and identification with the active male subject position has largely gone unchallenged. It is through some of his female characters and their relationship to food, I argue, that Hitchcock in fact carved out a space for feminine identification. The notion that food may be invested with love, goodwill, and good faith is one that Hitchcock's female characters embrace much more often than his men. In this regard, I would suggest that Hitchcock identified with many of his female characters, even though he rarely, if ever, professed such an identification. His biographer John Russell Taylor makes this point more forcefully, stating, "it was actually his heroines that he identified with." Naturally, because of the strongly gendered division of labor that structures our culture, it is not surprising that women, more often than men in his films, took on the role of preparing and providing food. But there are poignant moments—such as Constance's liverwurst, Alicia's roasted chicken, Blanche's hamburger—that witness his strong female characters expressing passion for food as well as romance in a manner that was resonant with Hitchcock's own sense of pleasure. And these female characters become more likable and accessible to the spectator through their expressed passion.

Of course, this love of food is not restricted to Hitchcock's female characters. One wonderful example of a male character strongly motivated by the pursuit of culinary pleasure—for whom Hitchcock held great fondness—is *Strangers on a Train*'s Bruno Anthony (Robert Walker). Hitchcock would often aver some variation of the idea, "The stronger the villain, the stronger the picture," and his premier example of this adage was always *Strangers*. He would repeatedly attest to his preference for the villainous Bruno character over the blander, more predictable everyman Guy Haines. In his famous interview, Truffaut remarked that Walker "gives a rather poetic portrayal; he's undoubtedly more attractive. There is a distinct impression that you preferred the villain," to which Hitchcock quickly replied, "Of course, no doubt about it."[31] Charlotte Chandler insightfully remarks, "Food frequently appears in Hitchcock films, and even when it seems not to serve a purpose, it helps define the characters." She strengthens this assertion with Hitchcock's own take on consumption and characterization.

> Preferences in food characterize people. I have always given it careful consideration, so that my characters never eat out of character. Bruno orders with gusto and an interest in what he is going to eat—lamb chops, French fries, and chocolate ice cream. A very good choice for train food. And the chocolate ice cream is probably what he thought about first. Bruno is rather a child. He is also something of a hedonist. Guy, on the other hand, shows little interest in eating the lunch, apparently having given it no advance thought, in contrast to Bruno, and he merely orders what seems his routine choice, a hamburger and coffee.

This self-assessment, of course, echoes the argument put forth earlier in the chapter that Hitchcock's precise attention to cinematic food and consumption was symptomatic of his unwavering commitment to a material realism that governed his films. His exemplum here also reveals that he formed cinematic attachments to characters who shared his sensibilities regarding the importance of pleasure, specifically culinary pleasure, in their lives. In his view, identification and emotional attachment to a character are predicated less on an adherence to strict moral decision-making and more on the recognizably human pursuit of pleasure and satiety. Were it otherwise, we would feel unqualified repulsion for Bruno based on his actions, and our full support would rest with the superficial do-gooder Guy. Yet our attachments are more complicated, more interesting, and Hitchcock was aware of pleasure's amoral and magnetic properties.

Food and sex are imbricated in Hitchcock's cinema, of course, in less savory ways as well. Just as culinary and sexual pleasures may be synergistic and mutually elevating, they may also, in their simultaneous circulation, effect a dehumanizing objectification. Specifically, the equation of women with food may emphasize qualities such as disposability, spoilage, and frivolity. The woman-as-food metaphor may run the gamut from seemingly benign, if tasteless, such as in *North by Northwest*, when Thornhill sends candy to a woman, inscribing it, "Something for your sweet tooth, baby, and your other sweet parts," to deeply dysfunctional and malicious, as in the dark metaphoric explorations of *Frenzy*. Tania Modleski has offered a definitive and wonderful account of the role of food and consumption in her chapter "Rituals of Defilement: *Frenzy*." In her articulation of the problematic woman-as-food metaphor, we may see in *Frenzy*'s "brutality toward women still one more indication of the need expressed throughout Hitchcock's works to deny resemblance to—absorption by—the female."[32]

What is more, "the identification of male with devourer and female with devoured" is martialed to "negat[e] the imagined ability of the female to absorb the male."[33] To be sure, the film invites a rather strictly gendered view of the consumer and consumed, most pronouncedly in the rape and murder of Brenda Blaney (Barbara Leigh-Hunt), before which Bob Rusk (Barry Foster) taunts her, "You know, in my trade, we have a saying; we put it on the fruit. 'Don't squeeze the goods until they're yours.'" Shortly thereafter, Rusk makes her "his," and demonstrates it by strangling her. That conceit, combined with the disposal of third victim Babs in a sack of potatoes, builds a strong metaphoric link not simply between food and murder, but among food, murder, and women. Thus, the confluence of the culinary, the carnal, and the coital do not unconditionally produce a palatable circuitry of pleasure.

Hitchcock weaves and entwines the signifiers of food and murder in provocative ways that are not always as estranging and degrading as witnessed in *Frenzy*, and he shapes these entanglements in the service of suspense and comedy equally. In *Blackmail*, Alice, having slain her would-be rapist with a knife, later hears the word "knife" interminably in her head, and the audience hears the word expressed impressionistically, as it is spoken at the breakfast table. She clutches the bread knife shakily as the word knife repeats, until, seized by guilt, she flings the knife across the dining room. Correspondingly, in the reverse, *Sabotage* eight years later contains a dinner scene in which Mrs. Verloc cuts a side of beef before using the carving knife to kill her husband. (The killing-carving-carving-killing that structures *Blackmail* and *Sabotage* is a nice chiasmus formation.)

Toward the climax of *Suspicion*, characters discuss cadavers and vivisection as they probe the meat on their dinner plates; in *Notorious*, Grant and Bergman discuss the preparation of a chicken dinner while embracing with delectation. The murderers of *Rope* proudly serve dinner on a large chest that contains the fresh corpse of their missing dinner guest; Rupert (James Stewart), upon learning of their scheme, cries out, "Did you think you were god? Is that what you thought when you served food from his grave?" In *To Catch a Thief*, Robie informs his lunch companion Hughson that the woman who prepared their delicate quiche lorraine had "strangled a German general once without making a sound." Perhaps most comically, as *Frenzy*'s Inspector Oxford recounts the discovery of Babs Milligan's body to his wife, "The corpse was deep in rigor mortis. He had to break the fingers of the right hand to retrieve whatever they held," Hitchcock cuts to an extreme close-up of Mrs. Oxford's hand snapping a breadstick in half, producing a ludicrous image of transubstantiation.

In charting these various dramatic linkages among sex, food, and death, it becomes clear that a large portion of these connections are forged in one of Hitchcock's archetypal scenarios: the dinner table. For Hitchcock, the dinner table is a theater of sublimation, displacement, and condensation, where pivotal issues of power and knowledge are often ominously invoked, transformed, or re-submerged. It is perhaps at Hitchcock's dinner table that the disparity between the veneer of calm civility and the chaotic desperation aroused by the films' central conflict is most pronounced. The dinner table foregrounds the repressive mechanisms that have enabled the status quo and simultaneously suggests their strong potential for breaking down. In *Young and Innocent*, Erica Burgoyne (Nova Pilbeam) sits rigidly at the lunch table guarding her secret knowledge of alleged murderer Robert Tisdall's (Derrick de Marney) whereabouts as her brothers discuss the food that a man on the run would arm himself with. In *Shadow of a Doubt*, Mr. Newton and neighbor Herb Hawkins debate the finer points of a successful hypothetical homicide as young Charlie (Teresa Wright) struggles with the knowledge of her uncle's true identity as the Merry Widow Murderer. Lina Aysgarth (Joan Fontaine) of *Suspicion* sits in dread, contemplating the possibility that her husband Johnnie (Cary Grant) is planning her murder, as he tries to extract information from Isobel (Auriol Lee) and her brother about the existence of an untraceable poison.

Throughout Hitchcock's work, several paradigmatic moments of the dining room scenario emerge that illuminate the repressed or unspoken dynamics of the meal in question.

1 The soup course—(e.g. *Murder! Shadow of a Doubt, The Paradine Case*). Hitchcock occasionally uses the first course to show a character's lack of engagement in the ongoing meal. He singles out the character who is not sipping the soup as rapidly as the other, and frames them in a long take, often as they are listening to the exposition around them. The soup course is also useful from a practical perspective, as Hitchcock was reluctant to show characters chewing.

2 Buttering bread—(e.g. *Rebecca, Suspicion, The Paradine Case, Rear Window*). The act of buttering bread at Hitchcock's table often suggests careful deliberation. Visually, it summons several metaphors, such as "What side is your bread buttered on?" (questions of loyalty, identity, and obligation); "spreading it on thick" (acts of flattery, manipulation); "spreading oneself too thin" (again, loyalty, and self-preservation). Nurse Stella in *Rear Window*, while making Jeffries a sandwich, claims she will "spread some common sense on the bread," so that he may ask Lisa to marry him.

3 Carving meat—(e.g. *Sabotage, Suspicion, Notorious, Under Capricorn*). The one designated to carve meat at the table is often the one with the perceived upper hand (except in *Sabotage*, though Mrs. Verloc does, indeed, get the upper hand). The carving of meat several times accompanies talk of forensics, of investigation, of getting to the "meat" of the matter—the strongest example, of course, being *Suspicion*, as the carving visually figures Lina's search for the truth about her husband.

4 Close-up on hands—(e.g. *Suspicion, Spellbound, Notorious, Under Capricorn, I Confess*). While Hitchcock mostly uses medium and medium close-up shots in his dinner table sequences, he occasionally resorts to a close-up or extreme close-up, usually on a character's hands, to show nervousness, tension, and stress.

5 Moments of rupture—(e.g. *Shadow of a Doubt, The Paradine Case, Frenzy*). The dramatic tension generated by the unspoken anguish of one or more of the characters is frequently broken through a visual distraction: as mentioned earlier, the breaking of a wine or brandy glass, or the sudden verbal protestation of a character, followed by their exiting the dining room. These moments mark the successful return of the repressed, and indicate that the protagonist (usually) has reached their breaking point.

Michael Walker rightfully observes that, in Hitchcock's world, "Food is rarely simply a means of nourishment, and meals are rarely simply an occasion for eating."[34] He focuses his discussion of food and meals primarily on their elucidation of sexual dynamics of the married couple and finds, "Overall, then, meals are something of a battleground for Hitchcock's married couples. . . . In Hitchcock, [food] is more likely to focus [tensions, rather than relieve them]." I suggest that Hitchcock's meals provide insights into relationships far beyond the romantic dyad. At his dinner table, we are often privy to triangulations and group dynamics, platonic relationships, as well as adversarial ones. In all these cases, food, drink, and their consumption become clever and multi-tiered indices of unspoken, internal character development.

Hitchcock and the signifying food chain

> I'd like to try to do an anthology on food, showing its arrival in the city, its distribution, the selling, buying by people, the cooking, the various ways in which it's consumed. What happens to it in various hotels; how it's fixed up and absorbed. And, gradually, the end of the film would show the sewers, and the garbage being dumped out into the ocean. So there's a cycle, beginning with the gleaming fresh vegetables, and ending with the mess that's poured into the sewers. Thematically, the cycle would show what people do to good things. Your theme might almost be the rottenness of humanity.[35]

In the above quotation, Hitchcock was sharing his idea with Francois Truffaut for a film that never materialized. The conceit intrigued Truffaut, who responded, "The story is a perfect illustration of your approach to a film. You start by spelling out all the imagery and the eventual sensations; from there on, the over-all theme will emerge by itself. It could be a fascinating picture." Funnily enough, much of the short treatment he offered was simply a further literalization of the tropes that had dominated his work for fifty years prior. Contained in that précis, we may recognize the familiar Hitchcockian reverence of food for its aesthetic value; the recognition of food's many metaphorical expediencies; the notion of food's dual evocation of pleasure and regret, or disgust. The foregrounding of the cyclical nature of consumption and elimination may have been something of an innovation in respect to the Hitchcock oeuvre. Yet, the rhythms of life's cycles have been present in some forms in his entire body of cinema. Sadly, the emphatic privileging of the "rotten" aspects of the cycle seems to have preoccupied him more and more toward the end of his life.

A chapter, or even a book, could not exhaustively explore the semiotics of food, drink, and waste in the films of Hitchcock. There are countless other fascinating ways in which food functions to produce narrative and visual meaning and pleasure that have not been broached here. For example, food as an indicator of class difference, as a psychoanalytic exploration of plenitude and lack, as a commodity studded with various socioeconomic histories, as a marker of ecologies in flux—all of these topics could provide interpretive lenses for Hitchcock's work. In the above meditations, I hope to have articulated some of the important ways that Hitchcock's passions for, and preoccupations with, food translated into his cinema. While describing these acts of translation, I could not help but marvel at what seemed Hitchcock's overarching desire: to communicate and share *his own* desires with his audiences. He recognized that pleasure could be the closest thing to salvation in a frightening world, and his brilliant facility with the language of pleasure, both visual and verbal, rendered each piece of his cinema an act of love.

4

Appetite and temporality in *Rear Window*: Another aspect of voyeurism

Is there no change of Death in Paradise? Does ripe fruit never fall? Wallace Stevens, "Sunday Morning"

In the sixty years since its release, *Rear Window* (Alfred Hitchcock, 1954) has assumed its place in the canon of Hollywood romantic thrillers, and carved a lasting niche among film critics and theorists as one of the *ur*-texts for making claims about voyeurism, meta-cinema, the male gaze, and the patriarchal design of the cinematic apparatus. From the formalism of Robin Wood, to the structuralism of Christian Metz, to the psychoanalytic feminist theory of Laura Mulvey and Tania Modleski, to the explication of authorial reflexivity delivered in the work of Jean Douchet, in France, and in the works of Robert Stam and Roberta Pearson, in America, *Rear Window* has become a canonical text for teasing out the complicated relationships among power, gender, ethics, desire, and identification that constellate to account for the voyeuristic appeals of cinema.

The scholarship on *Rear Window* is fabulously diverse in approach and in large measure incredibly sensitive to the formal and psychological dimensions of the visual field, and how that field stages struggles for power, epistemological insights and problems, and contradictory enunciations of gendered ways of looking. While the available critical body of work on *Rear Window* is voluminous and contains innumerable critical methodologies, one thing that unites the majority of it is a focus on the critique of voyeurism as it engages a fantasy of male mastery and control over the scopic object. Whether or not grounded in the language of psychoanalysis, there is a tendency to describe textual (and sexual) relations between the desiring male subject (in the form of Jimmy Stewart's L. B. Jefferies) and the desired object of cinematic femininity, the "bearer of the look," as Mulvey would designate female positionality (in the form of Grace Kelly's Lisa Freemont, among others).[1]

This essay addresses an aspect of voyeurism that has rarely been fleshed out in regard to *Rear Window*, and one with which Hitchcock was eminently concerned. In addition to its being a beautiful visual essay on cinema, a meditation on the active and passive, subjective and objective, exploitative and ethical facets of the gaze, the film is also an intervention into the gaze as an insidious purveyor of the fantasy of the scopic object's fixity. This false notion of the fixity of the object of the gaze, which dovetails nicely with the much-discussed fantasy of mastery and control conferred on the desiring subject, may also be regarded as the fantasy of atemporality. Framed otherwise, the film problematizes the subject's apprehension of an object it perceives as frozen in time; it corrects the Keatsian endeavor to affix the object in time and space, to be fetishistically cherished in its imagined stasis.

In what follows, I hope to invigorate and enrich the critical discourse on *Rear Window* and the cinematic gaze through four central propositions. These contributions do not displace the primacy of voyeurism and the visual as fundamental tropes in both the film and the analysis of it, but complicate *how* and *what* voyeurism means in the context of *Rear Window*. Further, I intend to catalyze thinking about alternate, non-visual epistemologies dramatized in the film, and, perhaps most importantly, redirect critical attention of the film to Hitchcock's important interrogation of embodiment, far beyond the theoretical confines of the male subject's eye and the fragmented or fetishized female body. In the remainder of the essay,

1 I enlarge the frame of how voyeuristic pleasure circulates in the film; whereas most criticism focuses on L. B. Jefferies's relinquishing of a purely objectifying gaze (through which he succumbs to the illusion of mastery over the female object), and his adoption of an empathetic gaze (in which he comes to recognize an ethical relation to the newly subjectivized object), I propose another complementary narrative: Jefferies's progression from an objectifying gaze that fantasizes a static, atemporal object, to a gaze that recognizes the visual object as a dynamic subject in its own right, defined by change, consequence, and unpredictable growth.

2 I argue that, as much as it is a filmic essay on the visual, it is also a meditation on time, change, growth, and proportion.

3. I discuss the film as an examination of the ways a purely visual epistemology may be lacking, distorting, or even dangerous.
4. I suggest that, in delivering these object lessons on time and embodiment, Hitchcock consequently characterizes the film's women as unsophisticated (or at least comedic) in their understanding of the literal and figurative deployments of the body. This alignment of the feminine with the impeded understanding of bodily signification both undergirds the film's comedy and throws into relief Jeff's rehabilitated awareness of bodies that matter.

An eye for a stomach: The instructive case of Miss Torso

Hitchcock recalled the production and release of *Rear Window* fondly, sharing with Francois Truffaut in his famous series of interviews, "I was feeling very creative at the time, the batteries were well-charged."[2] Patrick McGilligan observes that, after reaching an all-time high weight of 340 pounds several years prior, Hitch had arrived at the all-time low weight of his adult life, 189 pounds, around the time of this shoot.[3] Consequently, his biographer John Russell Taylor reports, he had "seldom been happier."[4] Perhaps in this time of relative good health and stability, it was fitting that Hitchcock stand back and reflect on the rather tumultuous years of drastic flux with which he had become so familiar. At a conservative estimate, by 1954 he had gained and lost between 300 and 400 pounds, just since his arrival in Hollywood fifteen years prior. The drastic diet he had begun in 1942, resulting in a radical though temporary 100-pound weight loss, followed by lapses and recommitments throughout the decade and a half, no doubt produced a profound contemplation of his habits, his compulsions, his sense of discipline, and most of all, of his body, and all bodies, as a mercurial and unpredictable form. Because of the predominant focus on the visual field in existing scholarship on *Rear Window*, interpreting the film as an extended meditation on the changing nature of the body may seem an incredibly eccentric reading. Yet, in what follows, I hope to convey that a contemplation of the changing body is embedded in *Rear Window*'s narrative and in other spaces of its diegetic world, and that recognizing the vestiges of that contemplation enriches one's understanding of the film.

For very good reasons, most film criticism of *Rear Window*, whether psychoanalytically or structurally grounded, accepts the interpretation that Stewart's protagonist L. B. Jefferies can be convincingly regarded as either a double or a surrogate for the spectator, as well as for Hitchcock the director. In arguing for Jefferies-as-spectator, Jean Douchet remarks that the protagonist reproduces the conditions of the moviegoer at the theater; he or she is immobile (as is Jefferies, confined to his wheelchair) and he or she is in the position to look on at the lives of others, without having his gaze acknowledged or returned.[5] In Mulvey's account of visual pleasure, identification and desire, this arrangement confirms her assessment that the camera, the male protagonist, and the presumed male spectator converge to create the desiring male subject within the cinematic apparatus of classical Hollywood. In the account of Stam and Pearson, Stewart's Jefferies stands in for Hitchcock, as the film is fundamentally a reflexive exercise that foregrounds the theatrical and the performative aspects of cinema itself. In this optic, Jefferies is in the director's (wheel) chair; he is responsible for framing the stories of the neighbors he watches; he gives voice to their narratives and manipulates their images through his use of the binoculars and the telephoto lens. The rear window, they argue, provides a proscenium, and Jefferies "directs" the dramas of his neighbors, providing Lisa, Stella, and Doyle with the interpretive framework they require to make sense of the neighbors' actions.[6]

As convincing and satisfying a move that reading Jeff as cinematic surrogate is, suppose, for a moment, that we explore the possibility of another character's functioning as a hypothetical double for Hitchcock the director, not in place of Jefferies, but in addition. I ask that, for a moment, we look at the supporting character Miss Torso (played by Georgine Darcy) as a sort of Hitchcock double.

Superficially, a leggy blonde in her twenties, who is content to flounce around her studio in her underwear, and a "stout fellow" in his fifties, who never left his house without wearing a suit, may not seem to have much in common. One similarity between them is their shared status as visual spectacle. Miss Torso is a quintessential example of Mulvey's fetishized object of cinematic femininity, a figure primarily characterized by, in her words, "to-be-looked-at-ness."

Certainly within *Rear Window*, Grace Kelly is of primary scopic interest; she is the beautiful, charismatic leading lady. Miss Torso, however, is object *par excellence*. She performs constantly and suggestively (and also important, unwittingly) for Jeff's eager eyes; she barely registers a subjectivity and has almost no voice, save when defending herself from a drunk suitor at the door, and when her true love Stanley returns in the film's denouement.[7] Perhaps her status as exalted object is best revealed in the fact that Jefferies has named her for a part of her anatomy, giving her a fragmented, fetishized, and synecdochal relation to her own body.

Hitchcock himself experienced a definite sense of "to-be-looked-at-ness," albeit for very different reasons from Miss Torso and by different audience formations. Indeed, their curves may be differently shaped and differently valued, but they share in a similar self-consciousness and knowledge of their (differently) performative bodies. Hitchcock in fact draws on the absurdity and the humor of the notion that he might have something in common with a curvaceous woman. In the twenty-ninth episode of the third season of his *Alfred Hitchcock Presents*, entitled "Death Sentence," he facetiously boasts in his epilogue, "I received a very good job offer. An Italian actress needs a stuntman to take a bubble bath for her in her next picture. I was hired when it was discovered that the actress and I had the same measurements. In different places, of course." Thus, while I am not suggesting that Hitchcock consciously employed Miss Torso as a surrogate or a double for his directorial self, the linkage he made just two years later as a joke on his TV show, indicates that he had noted the similar but different status of the male fat body and the voluptuous female body as visual spectacle.

Also, very much like Hitchcock, Miss Torso is represented as having an unusual and remarkable relation to food. Critics have never commented on the fact that, most of the time she appears on screen, Miss Torso is filling her stomach. In the first five minutes of the film, we witness her dancing and eating simultaneously, as Jeff argues on the phone with his editor Gunderson about taking a plum photo assignment abroad. As he unrealistically—in denial of his immobility—pleads for a shot at covering a foreign coup, he watches Miss Torso dancing to the refrigerator while making a series of suggestive thrusts, then leaning into the icebox and pulling out a turkey leg and nibbling on it, before dancing back across the room. And then in a feat of voracious dexterity, she veritably "double-fists" her meal; while holding the poultry in one hand, she slathers butter (or a condiment like mayo) on a piece of bread, and then takes a big bite of the bread, before returning her attentions to the drumstick. When Stam and Pearson broach the topic of Miss Torso's strange habits, they discuss them in the context of her providing a sense of meta-theatricality to the film's mise-en-scene. They argue that each apartment across from Jeff fuels the metaphor of Jeff-as-director by playing out on his "cinema screen" a different film genre. They observe that the neighbors

> seem to have strayed directly from the various genres of the classical Hollywood film. Miss Lonelyhearts is borrowed from an earnest 1950s social realism film like *Marty;* Thorwald comes from a murder mystery; the dog couple comes from a domestic comedy. The songwriter belongs in a musical bio picture.[8]

They find, finally, that "Miss Torso belongs in an MGM musical, when not in 1950s soft core porn. A vulgar utopian, she transforms the quotidian—brushing her teeth, checking the refrigerator—into musical comedy-style song and dance."

While "vulgar utopian" may be an odd characterization of the dancing figure, their point is well taken that the visual comedy that she provides is rooted in the juxtaposition of the banal routines of daily life, with the *joie de vivre* of spirited choreography. What they fail to notice is the predominance of images of consumption that accompany her dancing. After this scene with the turkey leg, she is seen eating twice more—as she pulls leftovers from the fridge, and then later eats a sandwich while reading a novel (two kinds of consumption at once). Interestingly, Stam and Pearson mention both the MGM musical and "1950s soft core porn" as the genres that Miss Torso may represent to Jeff-the-director. Certainly her scantily clad, suggestive dances evoke sexual desire for Jeff, based on his reaction, and later, his friend Doyle as well. The addition of her "erotic eating" may come across as puzzling, or just plain funny.

Yet it is important to read these images in the context of Hitchcock's body of work. *Rear Window* is not the first film where Hitchcock has used food to suggest sexual appetite or arousal. In *Notorious*, we have the famous "chicken scene," where Bergman's Alicia and Grant's Devlin kiss and paw at one another, while discussing the chicken she will make for dinner that night. In *Spellbound*, Bergman again gushes at the memory of eating a liverwurst sandwich with Gregory Peck's John Ballantyne. So, perhaps Hitchcock here relies on the dual evocation of appetites—sexual and culinary. Yet, I would also like to explore another potential effect that the portrayal of dancing and almost compulsive eating may generate for the viewer, albeit with great subtlety.

A moment in the film that, to my knowledge, has never been given critical attention, but is absolutely worthy of focus, arrives a third of the way through the film. It is the morning after the murder of Anna Thorwald, and Stella is giving Jeff a therapeutic back massage. She scolds him for staying up all night in his wheelchair, and makes a forceful case for the desirability of Lisa Freemont as a mate. After she points out his unhealthy voyeuristic compulsion, their conversation follows:

Stella: What are you going to do when one of them catches you?

Jeff: Depends which one. Now, Miss Torso, for example . . .

Stella: You keep your mind off her.

Jeff: She sure is the "eat, drink, and be merry" girl.

Stella: Yeah, she'll wind up fat, alcoholic, and miserable.

Stella's witty retort seems like a throwaway, either spoken out of simple envy, or indicating that she is invested in the coupling of Jeff and Lisa. Yet, the turn of phrase is striking. In one stringent barb, Stella punctures Jeff's fantasy of his scopic object's fixity, by bringing her into the world of time and change. In her deflation of Miss Torso, she counters the mutually reinforcing fantasies of the voyeuristic gaze: not simply that the object of the gaze is somehow the property of and under control of the desiring subject, but that she is an object removed from time and consequence, eternally accessible, not subject to change or growth that would annihilate the fantasy.

Jeff's description of her as the "eat, drink, and be merry" girl obviously is an ellipsis of the maxim, "Eat, drink, and be merry, for tomorrow we die." The phrase is a conflation of two biblical passages, Ecclesiastes 8:15, "Then I commended mirth, because a man hath no better thing under the sun, than to eat, and to drink, and to be merry," and Isaiah 22:13, "Let us eat and drink; for tomorrow we shall die." It is an exhortation to live in the moment, discounting past and future, seeking pleasure in the moment without regard to consequence. And, of course, it calls for consumption. Miss Torso is eating, drinking, and dancing, in some combination, nearly every time the camera trains on her. Stella's insult lends Jeff's nicknaming her by her stomach even greater weight. Not only has she been named by a portion of her anatomy that has excited scopic interest, but in Stella's retort, the woman becomes not just named, but defined by, the spectacle of her supposedly growing torso; her fantasy-inducing body will give way to a woman who is "fat, alcoholic, and miserable."

Framing the Eat, Drink, and Be Merry Girl

2:50	Grabs coffee pot and bag of coffee; spoons coffee while doing barre exercises.
5:01	Goes to fridge, pulls out a turkey leg. Dances, with turkey leg in hand. Butters bread, takes a bite of it, then takes a bite of the turkey leg in her other hand.
15:58	Sets out bottles of liquor for cocktail party.
23:45	Serves drinks and hors d'oeuvres to three male party guests.
34:50	Struggles to keep a drunk suitor from entering. Goes to fridge, pulls out turkey leg and takes a bite.
45:54	Lies on stomach on bed, reading book; takes a large bite of a sandwich and brushes crumbs off her chest.
1:50:59	Greets true love Stanley at the door, embraces him, as they walk together to the fridge.

Stella's remark also has the rhetorical effect of countering the acts of hedonism with their purported consequences. She answers Jeff's observation, "Eat, drink, and be merry," with the parallel construction, "fat, alcoholic, and miserable." In doing so, she counters the fetishistic fantasy of the object—one defined by the ever-present and by pleasure—with the fantasy-rupturing description of a body defined by dynamism and consequence.

The juxtaposition of Jeff's fantasy with Stella's realism generates a compelling tension that was certainly operative in Hitchcock's own life. Ever the epicure, famous for his lavish dinners, champagne lunches, and love of ice cream, Hitchcock understood the pleasures of the moment and their future consequences. "Fat, alcoholic, and miserable" would be a reductive, mean-spirited, and in many ways inaccurate description of Hitchcock at fifty-four (although Spoto would paint that picture of him repeatedly in his sometimes unduly harsh *Dark Side of Genius*), but it definitely encapsulates the unfortunate incommensurability of the fantasy of the frozen moment with the reality of the body that accumulates the expense of those moments.

Besides providing visual pleasure for Jeff, and presumably the spectator, Miss Torso stands at the center of her own subplot. We watch her eat (see the table above), dance, and flirt with men who seem like potential male suitors. Jeff introduces Lisa to some of the objects of his bored spectatorship, including her. He quips, "You remember, of course, Miss Torso, the ballet dancer? She's like a Queen Bee, with her pick of the drones," as they watch her balance the attentions of three men at a cocktail party crowding her studio apartment. Lisa empathetically adds commentary, "She's doing a woman's hardest job—juggling wolves." When she steps out onto her balcony with one of the men, isolating him from the two jealous suitors inside, Jeff, perhaps with a degree of jealousy himself, cynically observes, "She certainly picked the most prosperous looking one," to which Lisa quickly retorts, "She's not in love with him, or any of them." When Jeff inquires how she knows this from afar, she strategically answers, "You *said* it resembled my apartment." In this response, Lisa evokes the idea that eligible men frequently populate her apartment, but that she is waiting patiently for Jeff to come around. Thus, the answer suggests the ease with which she could couple, but also her desire to wait for Jeff to acknowledge their fit as a couple.

Lisa, it turns out, is right; Jeff's narration of Miss Torso as eligible bachelorette is wrong. Miss Torso is not Circe after all, but Penelope, patiently waiting for the return of her love, while fending off suitors who do not measure up. The payoff of this story, of course, unfolds in the denouement, when Miss Torso's door opens to reveal Stanley, the scrawny, diminutive man of her dreams. Obviously, the moment is supposed to be humorous; she has put off men that are conventionally handsome, charming, and well-built, and it turns out that her preference is absolutely unconventional. In hugging Stanley, she dwarfs him. Her well-toned, slim yet curvaceous body suddenly becomes slightly ridiculous as it engulfs this small man in uniform. We are led to understand that he was even smaller when he left for army service, in her exclamation, "My, look what the Army's done for you!" Stanley responds, "The Army's made me hungry. What've you got in the icebox? Boy, it's good to be home!" at which point they walk to the refrigerator, arm in arm. Perhaps, then, we are to infer that Miss Torso has been eating to sublimate her desire until the homecoming of her romantic partner. His long-awaited return begins, though, not with a romp in the sack, but a snack. Miss Torso's connection to food and consumption is unbroken, even in the film's resolution. She is by no means "fat," as Stella had predicted, but she is still somewhat compulsively at the mercy of her stomach.

The original trailer of *Rear Window* introduces the audience to the key players of the film, of course, but also gives a cursory treatment of the neighbors—treatment that is occasionally misleading, as to their characters, and sometimes not at all what we find in the finished product of the film. Later, I discuss its portrayal of Miss Torso's downstairs neighbor, but here I wish to draw attention to what is said about her. In her segment, three men in expensive suits stand in her apartments, somewhat awkwardly, while she dances around them. The scene is likely supposed to introduce her habit of dancing in her apartment, and her task of entertaining suitors. The voice-over comments, "Miss Torso, the body beautiful! That is, viewed from a distance!" The trailer's script is not particularly well-written, and this description is particularly curious. It either implies that she is *not* beautiful when viewed up close, or that it is unsafe to view her up close. If it is, in fact, not "safe" to gaze at her except from afar, the implication perhaps is that she is spoken for, and a man who expresses desire for her is in for confrontation. Of course, this description may be intended to generate a buildup for the ultimate reveal of Stanley at the film's end, whereupon we realize that the threat was minimal all along.

This interpretation of Miss Torso's function in the meta-narrative of visual fantasy, as an object lesson in understanding a scopic object as mobile, dynamic, not fixed in time, or outside of it, expands our idea of the assumptions that undergird the voyeuristic gaze. A literary example of this aspect of the male gaze can be found in Zora Neale Hurston's great novel *Their Eyes Were Watching God*. In the opening of the novel, beautiful Janie Crawford has returned home after a long time away from her village, and the onlookers at her arrival exhibit jealousy and skepticism upon her return. Hurston humorously depicts the divergent reactions of the men and women present:

> The men noticed her firm buttocks like she had grapefruits in her hip pockets; the great rope of black hair swinging to her waist and unraveling

> in the wind like a plume; then her pugnacious breasts trying to bore holes in her shirt. They, the men, were saving with the mind what they lost with the eye. The women took the faded shirt and muddy overalls and laid them away for remembrance. It was a weapon against her strength, and if it turned out of no consequence, still it was a hope that she might fall to their level some day.[9]

The image here of Janie's return is an image to be mentally affixed, for the voyeuristic pleasure of the men and for the condescending, and defensive, judgment of the women. It recalls the action of a snapshot—though cameras were scarcely available in the novel's all-Black Florida town of Eatonville in the 1930s. The image, fixed in time and space, produces pleasure through its imagined stasis of the object represented. Hurston suggests a masturbatory aspect of the frozen image, the one the men "[save] with the mind." In contemporary parlance, we often hear one (usually a woman) say to someone (usually a man) who has been gazing too intensely or too long, "Take a picture; it will last longer." The deflection suggests that a snapshot will serve the same purpose, that a static representation of the one gazed on would stand in for the real body, and exist as an object long after the person is out of sight.

It is of particular importance that Jeff is a photographer by avocation. Stam and Pearson remark on the relevance of his profession to the creation of the motif of Jeff-as-director. As mentioned above, the film as a meta-commentary on film and the cinematic apparatus relies on the depiction of Jeff-as-Hitchcock, in his orchestration and narration of the images of the neighbors, and through his aesthetic manipulation of them, through light, angle, and framing. Stam and Pearson astutely mention, "The sequence of slides that Jeff projects calls attention to the static photograph as the primordial point of departure for cinematic illusion." The photograph, they argue, is the "primordial point of departure," in that the nineteenth century saw the evolution of the photograph into motion pictures, by way of serial photography. I would argue, in addition, that the static photograph—the product of Jeff's art—is the premier sign of the impulse for the fantasy of object fixity that the gaze promises. Before we as audience are introduced to Lisa, we see her static image, first in ghoulish negative (tellingly, the one that Jeff has framed), and then the positive print. Thus, Jeff trades in static images, and exhibits a comfort in images that are either static or remote (seen through binoculars or telephoto lens), a comfort he does not feel with people, particularly women, up close.

Cinema as a medium acts on us by involving us with the tension between the static and the kinetic. Filmic narrative is obviously dynamic; in classical narrative, we watch characters progress and change over time. Yet, the technology is one of stasis and object permanence. Like opening a novel, each scene we watch unfolds in an eternal present, no matter how many times we watch it. The medium "film" itself is named for the material film stock that captures the static images, and then relays them to us in rapid succession. As an artifact, a reel of film is a collection of static images that generate our own fantasies of object fixity; Scarlett O' Hara, Ninotchka, Stanley Kowalski, and Lisa Freemont will always appear to us affixed in their youth and beauty, occupying the present, bodies outside time and consequence.

The idea of the movie still even heightens this sort of temporal fetishization we enjoy from cinema. The images are still, in the sense of being motionless, and also occur *still*, in the sense of "even now," a beacon of sameness and consistency in a world of unpredictable growth and change. Hitchcock clearly understood the pleasures of the fantasy of fixity, and yet recognized that good cinema had to challenge the fantasy by reminding us of the dynamism of humanity and the extra-diegetic world.

Hitchcock's aesthetic of rupturing the fantasy of atemporality can be glimpsed in all of his films, even the light romantic and comedic ones, in his refusal to end any of his pictures with an un-ambivalent "happily-ever-after." Even in the attainment of coupledom, something always looms that could prove to be the union's undoing. In *Notorious*, Devlin and Alicia are reunited, but she has been poisoned and may not live. In *To Catch a Thief*, John Robie and Frances admit their love for one another, but the presence of the mother-in-law promises trouble. Even in *North by Northwest*, the train may have entered the tunnel, but Roger and Eve still have to contend with the deceptive conditions under which they met. *Rear Window* is no different. At the end of the film, Jeff is doubly casted (and doubly castrated, as many critics would have it), and Lisa is now wearing the "pants." And, of course, she will always prefer a fashion magazine to a travel guide.

Jeff's insistence on the static extends beyond his professional embrace of the static image and the distant object. He fears change in several contexts. He argues with Lisa that they "keep things *status quo*." When Gunderson castigates him for saying that women nag, reminding him that, in the contemporary idiom of gender equality, women "discuss," he retorts, "Maybe in the high-rent district they discuss; in my neighborhood they still nag." Jeff evokes empiricism to deny the existence of change. He even resists Lisa's replacing his old cigarette case with a new one. When Stella laments the state of modern marriage for its clinical and "four-syllable-word" approach to intimacy, Jeff disingenuously evokes the pop psychology truisms of "progressing emotionally" and "emotional levels," not because he believes in them, but in order that he may not have to change and accommodate Lisa's plans for them. And, of course, Jeff equates marriage with the death of his bachelorhood and even, perhaps unconsciously, with death itself, as his quickness to imagine that the Thorwalds' quarrel has resulted in her murder indicates. All of these moments illustrate Jeff's gravitation toward the still and unchanging.

Yet *Rear Window*'s denouement abounds with the dynamism of life. The newlyweds that have been having constant sexual relations have not, in fact, been frozen in the "happily ever after"; their exciting honeymoon sex has lapsed into bickering and recrimination. Miss Lonelyhearts is lonely no more; the composer has finished his song and possibly found a mate; a new dog has replaced the murdered one; painters prepare the Thorwalds' apartment for the next tenant; Miss Torso has regained her partner. And, of course, Lisa has seized her chance. Time marches on. Even Hitchcock appears in the frame to remind us of that, as he winds the clock of the songwriter, in his eight-second cameo. Thus, Jeff has learned to mistrust (or, at least, subordinate) his fetishistic fantasy of the fixed object and to relinquish remaining static in his own life.

The temporality of everyday life is explored at length in *Rear Window*, not simply as a corrective to the fetishization of stasis, but also as a relative concept that varies among individuals who experience it rather differently. Time, in fact, is marked differently in each apartment. Anna Thorwald's time is divided by the meals that her husband brings to her in bed. The couple with the dog has developed a routine that begins with their alarm clock, and is punctuated by letting out the dog. Miss Lonelyhearts plots the time around romantic assignations—imagined or real—and spends the time in between either preparing for them, or lamenting their meaninglessness. The newlyweds pass time in rounds of lovemaking, in a seemingly endless repetition; the groom even shows weariness when, "like clockwork," he is called by his bride back to the scene of consummation. Thorwald's time, after he has murdered his wife, is incremented by smoking; the glowing tip of his cigar registers regularly. Jeff himself is at the mercy of the calendar that sluggishly makes its way toward the removal of his cast. On the night of the murder, his time becomes measured through Thorwald's trips out into the rain. Miss Torso's time passes through dances and frequent meals; the composer's, through drafts of the song slowly nearing completion. Between the beginning of the film and its end, we also acknowledge the time has changed through the thermometer, which first reads 94 degrees, then 70 degrees.

The problem of fit: Imagining change, growth, and proportion

The nucleus of *Rear Window*'s romantic plot is of course, whether Jeff and Lisa can achieve a "fit," whether their compatibility can be realized, despite their different priorities and visions of domestic life. The question of their romantic "fit" finds figurative elaboration in countless images and objects in the film's mise-en-scene. Instances arise periodically, in which Jeff, and at times the spectator, find objects and their proportions, their fit, puzzling or funny.

After Jeff has chastised Lisa for her incompatibility with the world of adventure travel, pointing out that she could never dress for the occasion, she brings to his apartment a garment bag she refers to as a "mock cross-over night case." As she opens it, teasing, "I bet yours isn't this small," the lock pops open on the tiny, compact case to reveal a fluffy robe, nightgown, and slippers. "Look at this. Isn't that amazing!" Jeff marvels, completely unprepared for the volume that could fit inside.

Also of comic proportion is the telephoto lens that Jeff produces to enhance his gaze at the neighboring apartments. He starts off the film watching with the naked eye; he then enlists Stella to grab his binoculars. After finding these unsatisfactory, he eventually retrieves the lens from his cabinet, and attaches it to the comically small body of his camera. The proportion of lens to body seems outrageous; Jeff has to balance the lens on his knee to extend the camera. The image is also funny in its phallic suggestion. It contains an intriguing mix of masculine and feminine signifiers. It seems to protrude rigidly from his body, like a phallus, and yet it is the piece that passively receives the penetrating image, which enters the inner chamber and imprints on the film stock. But the lens allows for a masculine intrusion upon the terrain toward which it is directed. If the lens is the "eye" to the camera's "body," it is absurd in its disproportionate fit.

Another instance of a strange or unusual fit is in the comic image of the neighbor's dog and its makeshift "elevator." The neighbors have worked out a system of letting the dog out without having to walk it themselves. The small dog fills up the entirety of a basket, connected to a rope and pulley, and when it is elevated by the couple above, the moment always elicits chuckles from the audience.

The question of fit becomes interesting to Stella as she gleefully "plays detective" alongside Jeff. Her discussion of size and fit, which will be explored at greater length in the chapter's final section, takes the form of contemplating the logistics of Thorwald's crime. In addition to deciding that the bathtub must be the only place the corpse would fit to be dismembered and drained, she and Lisa quibble over what body parts would fit in the small garden plot that they later excavate. Stella's curiosity about "fit" comes back to haunt her, when she learns of the head in the hatbox across the way.

The fit of characters' clothes also draws the eye and makes comment on their situations. Whereas the snugness of Miss Torso's garments draws attention to her status as an object of Jeff's desire, the snugness of Thorwald's clothes evoke *pathos*—the notion that he is uncomfortable with his size, and possibly without the money for a new wardrobe. Thorwald's fat, which shows in his protruding shirt buttons, also may suggest for Jeff that the man has grown flabby and impotent in his servile role in marriage. On the other end of the spectrum, the songwriter perhaps signifies as "starving artist" through the ill-fitting looseness of his clothes and the necktie that has been deprived of any slack. The roominess of Jeff's pajamas also lies in stark contrast to the professional tailored lines of Lisa's garments, visually reproducing their difference in temperament, formality, and compliance with convention.

The variation in size of all the neighbors of Jeff's apartment perhaps contributes to this visual exploration of proportion and fit. In his interview with Hitchcock, Truffaut thoughtfully explains what he perceives as the function of the neighbors.

> Everything [Jeff] sees across the way has a bearing on love and marriage. There is the lonely woman with no husband or lover, the Newlyweds who make love all day long, the bachelor musician who drinks, the little dancer whom all the men are after, the childless couple who dote on their little dog, and, of course, the married couple who are always at each other's throat.[10]

Thus, when Jeff gazes at the apartments across the way, he is contemplating what his future may look like, in terms of love and relationships. The variation of the sizes of character may be another source of contemplation of his future. As mentioned, Thorwald, the henpecked husband, is the fattest of the cast. Miss Torso's downstairs neighbor, the sculptress, has a pear-shaped body. The newlyweds are of average stature. Miss Torso, of course, is the film's "body beautiful." Miss Lonelyhearts carries a slightly thin build. And the songwriter is quite thin and haggard; only Stanley, Miss Torso's long-awaited beau, proves to be more diminutive. The selection of very diverse body types may not have been a consciously motivating factor in the casting decisions of *Rear Window*; yet the variation plays nicely into the mise-en-scene as it is visually engaged with notions of growth and change.

Another source of puzzlement for Jeff regarding size and change arises when he is comparing slides he has taken of the courtyard garden. He asks Lisa to view two slides, hoping she will be able to remark the same change that he himself observes. In explaining the change to her, he alternates the slides, deliberating, "There's one important change. Those two yellow zinnias aren't as tall as they used to be. Since when do flowers grow shorter?" It is this absurdity in the notion of a flower's growing in the wrong direction that leads Jeff to the conclusion, "Something's buried there."

When seeing is not believing

In addition to its dramatization of the ways that the gaze may plague the seeing subject with false ideas about its relation to the object and the meanings of that reductively dichotomized relationship, *Rear Window* also demonstrates ways in which purely visual epistemologies may fail to provide nuanced or balanced interpretive frameworks. Stam and Pearson pronounce the visual field as the central epistemological tool of the film, elicited in its very title.

> [The title] evokes the diverse "windows" of the cinema: the cinema/lens of camera and projector, the window in the projection booth, the eye as window, and film as "window on the world."

They also cite Christian Metz, who contends that cinema "demands an immobile secret viewer who absorbs everything through his eyes" and attains, through primary identification with Jeff and his instruments of visual magnification, "the illusory god-like power of the 'all-perceiving spectator'." It is interesting to note the slippage that occurs between vision and perception, the presumptive move from absorbing "everything" through the eyes, to becoming the "all-perceiving spectator."

Clearly, perception, and the knowledge it produces, exists outside the visual, and the film makes us aware that over-reliance on visual information may be not only misleading, but possibly dangerous. As Stella enters Jeff's apartment for the first time in the film, she tells him that in ancient times, the penalty for Peeping Toms was the receiving of a red-hot poker in the eye. Soon after, Stella boasts to Jeff that she has a "nose for trouble," launching into her story about having predicted the stock market crash on the basis of the CEO of General Motor's toilet habits. Later, after Jeff has pressed his luck in asking for his binoculars, she reaffirms, "Trouble. I can smell it." The film, in fact, makes many references to other organs besides the eye. Besides Stella's nose, Lisa inquires about Jeff's leg, and then his stomach, to which he replies, "Empty as a football," which may reference the missing stomach of the sculptress's piece across the way. Obviously, we have the reference to "Miss Torso," and various comedic references to dismembered body parts.

Robin Wood, in his pioneer work on *Rear Window*, discusses the spectator's alignment and identification with Jeff, noting that the identificatory bond with him is yoked to our seeing and knowing what he knows. Wood claims, "With one brief exception (when Jeffries is asleep, we see Thorwald, the murderer, leave his apartment with a woman), we are allowed to see only what he sees, know only what he knows."[11] The moment Wood mentions is an important one; had Jeff seen Thorwald and the woman in black exit, he would have had earlier confirmation that he was in cahoots with someone to commit murder. Yet, Wood's observation, apart from making this same conflation of seeing and knowing, also omits another important moment of the viewer's divergence from Jeff's visual field—one which most critics, in reiterating Wood's observation, also overlook. In one of the final scenes, just prior to the climactic arrival of Thorwald in Jeff's apartment, Jeff is scrounging for money that Stella may use to bail Lisa from jail. While they are thus engaged, the camera cuts to Thorwald's apartment, showing him leaving it and starting down the stairs, unobserved by Jeff. Obviously, this cut inaugurates another situational irony, making us privy to something that Jeff is not, and articulates his failure to see what almost costs him his life.

Stella's avowed "nose for trouble," skeptically regarded by Jeff, turns out to be accurate in this instance. Lisa, additionally, purports to have knowledge outside the purview of the gaze. She playfully offers to trade her "feminine intuition for a bed for the night." Jeff takes her up on the offer, but likely does not expect her "intuition"—more accurately, her knowledge of human nature and women's habits—to yield results. However, it is Lisa's conviction that Anna Thorwald would not leave on a trip without taking her wedding ring with her that moves their amateur investigation forward. Thus, the film evinces a sense of the frequent insufficiency of the visual to produce knowledge that is complete, accurate, and useful. At times, it suggests, the "gut" is worth listening to.

"I want *no* part of her": Women and the comedy of corporeal errors

As Stam and Pearson suggest, *Rear Window* narrates L. B. Jefferies's trajectory from a voyeur, preoccupied with the fetishistic, distancing, and vicarious aspects of the gaze, to an ethical neighbor who rejects his former passivity and gazes, not with narcissism, but with beneficent human interest. And, of course, as a corollary of this character growth, he transitions from a place of anxiety regarding Lisa and her marital intentions, to a space of appreciation of and affection for her, whereby he comes to prefer the woman in the flesh to the fetishized and fragmented woman of the fantasies engaged by his voyeurism. And hardly tertiary, he and Lisa, with the help of Stella and Doyle, solve a thoroughly satisfying murder mystery.

Hitchcock never created a taut and suspenseful thriller without the release valve of comedy. In his typical conscientiousness concerning the balancing and modulating of cinematic mood, he offers, "For me, suspense doesn't have any value if it's not balanced by humor. In the mystery and suspense genre, a tongue-in-cheek approach is indispensable."[12] Undoubtedly, *Rear Window* is recognized as one of Hitchcock's more enjoyable and engaging comedies, and the stuff of its comedy is usually attributed to the wonderful repartee of Stewart and Thelma Ritter, the wisecracking nurse who lovingly disciplines Stewart's romanticized loner into accepting and embracing Lisa as a mate. Using "homespun wisdom" and impassioned diatribes against "modern marriage," with all of its attendant psychologizing and clinical posturing, to loosen Jeff's attachments to bachelorhood and female fetish, Ritter's Stella is the comedic heart of the film.

Yet, Hitchcock employs other, less often acknowledged sources of comic relief to modulate the thriller's tone. He establishes a running joke about several of his female characters and their ineptitude in discerning the literal from the figurative, in their dealing with bodies both live and dead. More specifically, he uses the comic failings of Lisa, Stella, and the sculptress—identified in the trailer as Miss Hearing Aid—to speak with intelligence and insight about bodies, not only to periodically scale down the dramatic stakes of the thriller, but also to throw into relief Jeff's newfound sophistication regarding the importance of eschewing objectified bodies in favor of understanding bodies as subjects.[13]

Miss Hearing Aid is one of the minor neighbors depicted in the Greenwich Village apartment courtyard. She has three exchanges with neighbors and passersby, and is never acknowledged or spoken to by Jeff, although his (and our) glance trains on her sporadically. We see through her activity that she, like many of her neighbors, is an artist. Throughout the film, she is at work on a sculpture; interestingly, it is of a torso—Jeff's name for her upstairs neighbor—without a head and without a stomach. Thirty-six minutes into the film, an ice man passes her by, lugging a large block of ice, and inquires, "What's that supposed to be, Ma'am?" "It's called, 'Hunger!'" she proudly responds. And with that, the camera tilts upward to Miss Torso, who is practicing dance steps and who, in contrast to most shots of her, is not eating.

The moment is funny, because Miss Hearing Aid's piece is abstract, yet it evokes a gross literalization of the body. Instead of depicting hunger as also a psychological or emotional state, it is, in her rendering, purely an absence of stomach. In her bohemian surroundings, populated with artists of all kinds, she has produced a work of perhaps embarrassing literalness and little subtlety. Obviously, artistic appreciation is subjective, and it would be difficult to predict exactly what the reception of this piece would be in 1954 Manhattan, though I can report in contemporary screenings of the film, the moment usually evokes laughter, and taken together with the other key moments in which she is represented—when she is told to "Shut up" by Thorwald as she tries to give him advice about over-watering his garden, and later, when she is shown sprawled out on her lawn chair dozing in the film's denouement—the intention of her character seems to be a predominantly comedic one.

In the film's theatrical trailer, the voice-over accompanying Miss Hearing Aid hard at work pronounces, "He calls her 'Miss Hearing Aid,' an artist of a very odd and strange art." As the voice-over speaks, the camera frames her face through the empty space where the stomach of the sculpture would be located. The clumsy, literal quality of her piece, entitled "Hunger," perhaps draws attention to her own zaftig body, particularly as it reads in concert with her svelte ballet dancer neighbor. That her own appearance is of a "well-fed" woman ironizes the concrete-abstract artistic statement of her piece. Thus, the humor of her character emanates from her confused or shallow conception of representations of the body—a conception of which Jeff is largely "cured" by the end of the film.

The banter of Lisa and Stella regarding bodies and corpses constitutes another source of comic relief. Stella's working-class status seems to be reflected in her "unladylike" remarks and her refusal to use euphemism in discussing the hypothetical murder across the courtyard. In the first instance of her coarseness, Stella has just brought Jeff his breakfast of coffee, toast, butter, jam, fried eggs, and crispy bacon. Chewing on a piece of toast just behind his wheelchair as Jeff looks out the window toward the Thorwalds, she inquires, "Where do ya suppose he cut her up?" and answers her question before he has a chance to: "Of course! The bathtub! That's the only place where he could wash away the blood." Her bluntness causes Jeff to spill his coffee, and this indelicacy, not just a signifier of working-class manners (she earlier prefaces a remark to Jeff by saying, "Mr. Jefferies, I'm not an educated woman"), also elicits a chuckle because of her insistence in remarking on the literal and distasteful logistics of the crime.

Later, before Stella and Lisa embark on their mission to dig up the garden to find damning evidence of Thorwald's crime, their exchange plays for comedy.

> Jeff: He's cleaning up the bathroom walls.
>
> Stella: Must have splattered a lot. (Lisa gives her a disapproving glance.) Why not? It's what we're all thinking. . . . He's got to clean up those stains before he leaves.
>
> Lisa: Oh, Stella! Your choice of words!
>
> Stella: Nobody ever invented a polite word for a killing yet.
>
> The upper class sensibility that Lisa's protestation is meant to suggest contrasts nicely with Stella's working-class directness. Later in the scene,

after they have used the viewmaster to look at the changing height of the flowers, we witness the following exchange:

Jeff: Something's buried there.

Lisa: Mrs. Thorwald!

Stella: You haven't spent too much time around cemeteries, have you? Mr. Thorwald could scarcely put his wife's body in a plot of ground about one foot square, unless of course he put her in standing on end, and then he wouldn't need a knife and saw. No, my idea is, she's scattered all over town, leg in the East River . . .

Lisa: Oh, Stella.

The dialogue reads as comic not just because of Lisa's (and perhaps also Jeff's) repeatedly offended sensibilities, but also because in retrospect, Stella's remarks, however "off-color," are correct. In the film's resolution, as Thorwald gives his confession to the police, the cop who has taken him into custody tells Doyle, "Thorwald's ready to take us on a tour of the East River."

The above exchange is funny also because it instantiates a round of jokes about dismemberment, that read as humorously callous, and also rest on a sense of play between the literal and figurative body. As the female sleuths are collecting evidence of Mrs. Thorwald's demise, Lisa calls on Stella to confirm her feelings about women's habits with jewelry. When she asks Stella if she would ever leave home without her wedding ring, Stella vows, "The only way anybody could get that ring would be to chop off my finger." Stella's avowed devotion to her ring as a guarantor of her married identity is also accompanied by an unintentional reference to Anna Thorwald's possible dismemberment.

While the two women conspire to dig up the garden—as Jeff hilariously sits by in passive disbelief over their courageous determination—Lisa voices her approval of the plan: "Why not!" she declares, "I've always wanted to meet Mrs. Thorwald." The line shows that Lisa has sloughed some of her daintiness and is ready to proceed with a plan that may entail her encounter with a corpse. Lisa's expressed desire to "always [wanted to have met] Mrs. Thorwald" is both hyperbole—she only heard of Mrs. Thorwald forty-eight hours earlier—and a joke that confuses a social encounter with the living, with a macabre encountered with a likely dismembered corpse. Thus, the joke feeds on her surprising callousness and the idea that she may not have properly understood the gravity of her situation, let alone Anna Thorwald's.

Furthering the idea that the two women have taken on a perhaps foolhardy zeal for playing detective—foolhardy in that Lisa almost loses her life in the adventure, at the hands of Thorwald—their reaction to the reservations of

Jeff, who is less enthusiastic about their impending dig, comically depicts a gender role-reversal. Lisa brushes off Jeff's worried admonition, "Jeff, if you're squeamish, just don't look." The line draws laughs because of its intimation that Stella and Lisa are better equipped to deal with the darker side of the mystery than Jeff is. Lisa's advice, "Don't look," puts a comic spin on the whole concept of the male gaze with which the film is seemingly invested. Effectively, Lisa implies that Jeff's gaze is hardly one of mastery or control; in fact, the gaze may overpower or frighten him, as Lisa would have it. While Lisa at this moment seems to usurp the position of gazing subject, her imperiled circumstance in the following scene suggests that the bravado of her and Stella was unwarranted. The endangerment of Lisa, and subsequently Jeff, retrospectively belies their "tough talk" and the jokes they crack that play on the literal and figurative nature of the body.

The scene of Thorwald's capture contains the crowning joke of this comedic thread that evokes literal and figurative bodies, and particularly the allusions to dismemberment. When the arresting officer informs Doyle that Thorwald dug up the contents of the garden when the dog got too nosy and placed them in the hatbox in his closet, we are of course led to assume that the contents are in fact Anna Thorwald's head (another implicit reference to objects that *fit* in a container). Doyle glances at Stella and jokingly asks, "Want to look?" whereupon Stella retorts, in the final line of the film, "No, thanks. I don't want any part of her."[14] Clearly Stella intends to say, "I don't want any part of it [the macabre discovery waiting in the hatbox]," but her slip again evinces thoughts of dismemberment, her unwillingness to confront a fragment of Anna Thorwald, a "part of her." The camera fades out as the mistake registers on her face. Her blunder caps the climactic scene and seals the capture of the murderer with an air of absurd levity. Again a woman has been comically impolitic and "wrong" about bodies. It is a difficult moment to hash out in terms of a feminist reading—as are so many in this film—but despite the jokes made by and about women concerning embodiment, for me, it still registers as a sign that the film's women are ready to deal with bodies, whereas Jefferies has only been prepared to trade in images.

Time, change, and ambivalence

In his poem "Sunday Morning," Wallace Stevens depicts a woman's religious questionings. She has remained at home on a Sunday morning, preferring her own meditations on life and beauty to the sermons available to her in a church. The poem beautifully portrays her grappling with the question of immortality; it is sympathetic to her desire for a transcendent realm, beyond the strictures of time and change: "She says, 'But in contentment I still feel/The need of some imperishable bliss,'" to which the poetic speaker responds, "Death is the mother of beauty; hence, from her/Alone, shall come fulfillment to our dreams/And our desires."[15]

The woman's frustrated desire for "some imperishable bliss" approximates for me the appeal of the voyeuristic gaze, which bestows the comforting fantasy of an object's constancy or fixity. In a world defined by change, unpredictability, and, in the final analysis, death, the desire for an object that exists outside of time, not subject to consequence or decay, is perfectly understandable. The poetic speaker's gentle counter, "Death is the mother of beauty," suggests that the beautiful is predicated on change, that our apprehension of beauty is grounded in the knowledge of its evanescence. It is this relinquishing of the fantasy of fixity that *Rear Window* narrates. Embracing humanity in its dynamism and even its unpredictability becomes a salutary alternative to the fetishization of a desired object and the stasis it seems to promise.

Hitchcock, in his own experience of corporeal change, marked by triumph and failure, and ultimately acceptance, clearly had an ambivalent relation to change and growth. His construction of visual pleasure in *Rear Window*, and for that matter, in all of his films, certainly relies on the economy of the male gaze. Under his direction, the cinematic apparatus operates at full tilt, and the objectification of women feeds this machinery of desire. Yet, it is important to recognize the moments where he undermines the workings of this patriarchal design. Using Stella as a mouthpiece and Miss Torso as exemplum, he inflects his visual text with the suggestion that fantasies of control and mastery, and their attendant fantasies of atemporality and stasis, are eminently pleasurable, yet ultimately incommensurate with human connection. While on one hand, Jeff's acquiescence to Lisa's monogamous desires at the end of the film may constitute a surrender to the normative and coercive patriarchal plot, it also signals, perhaps, a willingness to value the organic change and unpredictability a real woman promises, over a fantasmatic embodiment of stasis that will eventually collapse on itself.

5

Childhood and the challenge of fat masculinity

I have rather a placid personality and I think I take after my mother in that respect. We both have what used to be called the cottage-loaf figure—a big oval, and on top of that is stuck a smaller oval.[1]

I received a very good job offer. An Italian actress needs a stuntman to take a bubble bath for her in her next picture. I was hired when it was discovered that the actress and I had the same measurements. In different places, of course.[2]

As we witnessed repeatedly in Chapter 1, Hitchcock was no stranger to poking fun at his weight, whether in an interview, a guest column, a speech, a press photo, or on his weekly TV shows. The fat humor he so often deployed, I have argued, served to diffuse and deflect the very real anxieties and depressive feelings he had regarding his weight and his inability to maintain control over it. In the two self-deprecatory quotes provided above, we witness a very rare variety of Hitchcock's fat joke—one that likens his body to a woman's. In the first, he claims his ample pear shape as an inheritance from his mother. In the second, he portrays his body as having an inappropriate or misplaced voluptuousness. The rarity of remarks like those above in his repertoire of self-deprecating humor brings me to the focus of this chapter.

In addition to his portly figure, Hitchcock embodied several other traits that ran conspicuously counter to the hegemonic signifiers of heterosexual manliness, particularly in 1940s and 1950s America: his Englishness would cause him in many contexts to be read as "effete," and his immaculate, dandy-like habits of hygiene and dress did nothing to obscure that reading. In addition to these potentially suggestive facets of his public persona, he was a self-confessed sexual innocent, mystified by the motives and meanings of femininity, and he was, above all, a sophisticated artist ensconced in a profession populated by the more expressively inclined. Hitchcock's artistic genius certainly did not exempt him from feeling the compulsory demands of gender conformity and masculine identity. He may have stood apart in his exceptional talent, but he desperately sought a life of normalcy and stability, and the sine qua non of his assured validation as "normal" rested in his role as husband and father of a traditional nuclear family.

In this chapter, I suggest that, just as Hitchcock's fat humor depressurized the "open secret" of his fatness, it also demonstrated an anxiety that his fatness may have read as effeminacy or embattled masculinity. In what follows, I examine these anxieties and discuss the various strategies, both inside and outside of his films that he employed in order to assuage or lessen the insecurities so firmly planted in his self-image and public perception. In particular, I engage with his construction of public persona, the filmic and extra-filmic characterizations of his relationship to children. In forging these connections between his experience of fatness and the remedies he sought to forestall the perceived questioning of his manhood, I produce an account of how Hitchcock's vulnerabilities surrounding childhood found their way into, and fundamentally marked, his cinema.

"You'll outgrow it": Hitchcock's youth

Hitchcock was born and christened Alfred Joseph Hitchcock, August 13, 1899, into a middle-class family of four, in Leytonstone; he was the youngest and final child, with an older sister and brother, seven and nine years older, respectively. Due to the considerable age gap between him and his siblings, Hitchcock recalls, "They didn't have much interest in me when I was growing up, so I had myself almost entirely to myself."[3] His homemaking mother was his primary companion throughout his childhood, and his father was an overworked greengrocer who seldom spent time with the family, apart from Mass on Sundays. The Hitchcocks were Catholic in a heavily Anglican environment, which gave them something of a self-perceived minority status.

Alfred was the only child in the family not to follow in his father's professional footsteps by adolescence. While his sister later gave up the business to marry, his father's namesake William Jr. took over the family business after the death of William Sr. at the age of fifty-two, in 1912. Hitchcock muses, "Perhaps I disappointed my father because I never showed any interest in his business and no inclination to follow him into it. I could not imagine how a wilted lettuce leaf could be of such concern to him."[4] Hitchcock in fact struggled to find much that filially bonded him and his father. He cleverly finds one point of intersection, however abstract: "My life's work has put me in a position not so different from that of my father—a speculator in perishables." Though he admits to feeling estranged from his father based on their lack of common interests, he nevertheless remembers, "Some of my happiest memories were on the rare occasions when my father took me with him to the countryside. He would buy a whole field of cabbages and that sort of thing."

The only other positive memories of his father that Hitch shared publically were the occasional family outings to plays and concerts. He observes, "My father never seemed carefree, except at the theater."[5] It is interesting to consider that Hitchcock chose as his avocation the one place that he experienced paternal harmony as a child. Hitchcock felt his father was emotionally remote, but powerful, nonetheless, and a good provider. One way in which he emulated his father was sartorially. He relates, "I remember my father going to work in a dark suit with a very starched white shirt and a dark tie. I never saw him when he wasn't clean-shaven. It wasn't for the cabbages. It was a matter of self-respect."[6] The description of his father's work apparel matches exactly the uniform he himself wore to his movie sets almost invariably for fifty years.

His other shared recollection was of his father's strong sense of discipline and order. Of course there is the ubiquitous tale Hitchcock told *ad nauseam*: that his father punished him at a very early age (five or six) by sending him to the local police station with a note asking the attending officer to lock up his son for a short period of time. If the story is true, the officer complied and ended the punishment with the now proverbial, "This is what we do to naughty boys"—an aphorism Hitchcock entertained putting on his tombstone. Apart from this apocryphal story that Hitchcock would often use to explain his aversion to policemen and other authority figures, his father William was, in the words of Donald Spoto, "a Cockney merchant who insisted on discipline, order, and simplicity in life as in diet."[7]

This paternal attitude toward strict diet was perhaps another cause of Hitch feeling estranged and considering himself, in his words, a "disappointment." From early on, Alfred enjoyed eating his mother's cooking and looked forward to visiting the local bakery. He recalls, "I was always given a free cookie or two. The bakery had the most wonderful aromas. Like perfume. Lemon Cake Number 5. Guerlain Ginger Biscuit."[8] Without a doubt, his mother and food were the primary signifiers of comfort and stability in his youth. He recalls that his mother would customarily require him each night to stand at the foot of her bed and report what he had done that day. We see this image of the son at the foot of the mother's bed used in *Notorious* with Alex Sebastian (Claude

Rains) and his emotionally demanding mother (Leopoldine Konstantin). And of course some version of the "Mama's Boy" is played out by Herb (Hume Cronyn) in *Shadow of a Doubt*, Bruno Anthony (Robert Walker) in *Strangers on a Train*, Norman Bates (Anthony Perkins) in *Psycho*, Mitch Brenner (Rod Taylor) in *The Birds*, and, less obviously, Bob Rusk (Barry Foster) in *Frenzy*.

Hitchcock attended a Jesuit-run school, where, he claims, his primary lesson was in fear. Less facetiously, he concedes that his schooling instilled in him an almost obsessive contemplation of right and wrong. Socially, however, school was not a productive place for him. In the words of Hitchcock's friend Charlotte Chandler, "His pudgy, overweight appearance, his lack of interest in the games the other children played, and little athletic ability isolated him and led to his development of more solitary interests." He recollects, "My mother was so consistently there for me. . . . [As a] homely, less popular child, I was forced to develop my interior self. . . . My private person, the real me, is a very shy person, not at all the public impression."[9] He recalls going home to his mother after being called "funny-looking" by a fellow student, and asking, "Do you think I look funny?" She offered the less than ideal consolation: "You'll outgrow it." In melancholy retrospect, he muses, "I didn't outgrow it. I just *outgrew*. No one wants to be fat. That's a universal."[10]

The misery of growing into his fat body clearly haunted Hitchcock as an adult. He reveals a heartrending nostalgia for a time in his youth before shame became inextricably entwined with food and eating. He laments, "I was able to enjoy [eating] because it was before I ever heard the word 'diet.' Plumpness in very small children was considered 'cute' and even a sign of good health. It reflected well on the parents and their prosperity, and showed they were taking good care of their child."[11] It is perhaps worth noting that, in this recollection of a time when his pleasures in eating were not socially stigmatized, he explicitly links his own consumption to his parents' social status. Implicitly, he seems to pine for this halcyon moment before his eating reflected poorly on himself and, by extension, his family. To his mind, the moment his body stopped signifying cuteness and health, it began to read as a shameful excess that set him apart from the other Hitchcocks. Thus he imagines his fatness to have produced "disappointment" that he projected on to his father.

Suffer little children: Hitchcock and cinematic childhood

Hitchcock's resentment of children who, by his accounts, were consistently antagonistic toward, or dismissive of, him in his youth, may partially explain his idiosyncratic uses (and abuses) of them in cinematic productions throughout his career. This hostility, however, does not (to this writer) fully account for the frequency and elaborateness with which he made disparaging remarks about children in his public life. Before I delve into the significance of children in his films, I examine the child as a trope in the construction of his public persona. In doing so, I suggest that Hitchcock strategically shaped the public's view of his attitude toward children. This purposeful manipulation of public sentiment was motivated not simply by juvenile animus, but by a need to fortify a sense of masculinity around his image. The anxieties he experienced around the question of his manhood were lessened by his crafting a persona that was resolutely unsentimental, anti-maternal, and dismissive of childhood's fragility or sanctity. In disavowing the touchy-feely associations with youth, he hoped to create a profile that conformed to the contours—stoic, inexpressive, unromantic, rational—of contemporary American masculinity.

In arguing for Hitchcock's drive to emulate and embody an acceptable or normative masculinity, I certainly do not mean to intimate that he approximated, or even desired to approximate, any version of *machismo*. He was clearly never the "cowboy" type (even if he *did* wear the hat in his *Psycho* cameo). Hitchcock had no illusions about the fact that he would never embody a masculine ideal. In fact, in some regards, he reveled in his unconventional masculinity, as witnessed in statements like, "I'm fortunate to be a coward, to have a low threshold of fear, because a hero couldn't make a good suspense film." Still Hitchcock recognized it was within his power to curtail or finesse certain associations that may have cast aspersions on his gender presentation and sexual identity. Thus, it was important for him to demonstrate that, even though he had his mother's "cottage-loaf" figure, he himself was not indulgent and motherly. His anti-child rhetoric was therefore deployed in the service of disavowing connections to the feminine and the maternal.

It is only natural that, as the "Master of Suspense" also responsible for two of the cinema's most successful horror films, Hitchcock was asked quite frequently about his own relationship with fear. And quite logically, he described fear's childhood origins. In one of his often-quoted meditations on the nature of fear, he says:

> Fear isn't so difficult to understand. After all, weren't we all frightened as children? Nothing has changed since Little Red Riding Hood faced the big bad wolf. What frightens us today is exactly the same sort of thing that frightened us yesterday. It's just a different wolf. This fright complex is rooted in every individual.[12]

In this statement, Hitchcock attempts to universalize the experience of acquiring fear, and he even frames his motivation for filmmaking as a sort of therapeutic means of alleviating the fears he took on as a child. Famously, he professed, "The only way to get rid of my fears is to make films about them."[13] In interview scenarios, he would habitually make reference to one of three childhood stories regarding the origin of his own fears. The first, of course, is the abovementioned encounter with the police, through which he claims to have acquired the fear of punishment, or fear of authority. Another story he would frequently employ was his memory of being left home alone by his parents who had been delayed on an errand. This anecdote obviously deals with the fear of abandonment. The third story he would tell dates back to his infancy when, while still in his crib, his mother surprised him with, "Boo!" Thus here, of course, originates the fear of the unexpected.

Apart from noting how his childhood provided the paradigmatic scenarios for the acquisition of adult fears, Hitchcock also played up a fear of children themselves in his publicity. He notoriously professed, "I am scared easily, here is a list of my adrenaline-production: 1. Small children; 2. Policemen; 3. High places; 4. That my next movie will not be as good as the last one."[14] His placement of "small children" at the top of the list of what scares him obviously is intended comically, yet it also gestures indirectly to Hitchcock's own experience of violence and indifference inflicted by his peers as a child. This list is echoed in a line delivered by Rupert Cadell (Jimmy Stewart) in *Rope*, though the sentiments are considerably harsher in this Hitchcockian mouthpiece. Rupert entertains the dinner party guests through what seems to be his usual tactic of *épater le bourgeois*. In his diatribe extolling the virtues of murder, he whimsically creates rules of etiquette for the act. He quips, "Knives may not be used on hotel employees. They are in the death-by-slow-torture category, along with bird lovers, small children, and tap dancers."

Obviously Hitchcock recognized that there was a fine line between the colorful and idiosyncratic expression of disdain for children and the unacceptably iconoclastic disregard for children's lives, and he would never risk voicing the degree of aggression contained in Rupert's speech, for fear of alienating the public. But the line still has intertextual resonance to an audience familiar with Hitchcock's reservations about children. Hitchcock's characterization of children as fear-inducing also finds its expression in *Frenzy* (1972), as two bystanders discuss the profile of a serial killer like the Necktie Strangler currently at large. One man warns his companion that psychotic murderers "appear as ordinary, likable, adult fellows, but emotionally they remain as dangerous children whose conduct may revert to a primitive, subhuman level at any moment."

Another instance in which Hitchcock distinguished himself as having a playful irreverence toward children can be found in the much-repeated anecdote about a child's viewing of *Psycho*. Hitchcock reports that a man wrote to him, telling him that he had taken his daughter to see Henri-Georges Clouzot's *Les Diaboliques* (1955), in which a woman is brutally stabbed to death in a bathtub. The man complained that after the film, his daughter would no longer take baths. Five years later, along came Hitchcock's *Psycho*, with its iconic shower murder scene, and now, the girl refused to take showers as well. When asked what he should do about his daughter's situation, Hitchcock reportedly sent back a laconic reply, "Send her to the dry cleaners." The remark is darkly funny, yet it also expresses a problem with the American enshrinement of childhood, whereby the policing of child hygiene and purity is a symptom of an ideology that casts the child in a cultural role of innocence to be protected at all cost, and, in the long run, fails to see the child in its human, less symbolic dimensions.

Hitchcock's frequently attacked adage "Actors are cattle" was among the most popular subjects of Hitchcock interviews. The director often made comments to the effect that actors' performances were less important to a film than the contributions of the director, and that performance could be shaped and manipulated in the editing room after a production had been committed to film. These remarks often painted Hitchcock as having an antagonistic relationship with his actors. This was usually not the case (with some notable exceptions), though Hitchcock enjoyed the inflammatory aspects of the notion. When asked if he *really* described actors as cattle, he usually offered the further joke, "I never said that. I said they should be *treated* like cattle." In another context, he playfully clarified, "Actors are children. They need to be petted and guided and should be patted on the head. Occasionally, they need a good spanking too."[15] In this only half-facetious gesture, Hitchcock manages simultaneously to disparage actors *and* children, linking their neediness and self-absorption. This clever rejoinder staged yet another opportunity to demonstrate his emotional disconnection from youth.

Two pieces of Hitchcock trivia that have circulated far and wide for many years warrant another look in the context of examining his inclination toward female dis-identification in his public persona. The first is his greatly publicized fear and loathing of eggs. Hitchcock brought his revulsion up in many interviews, always some riff on these images:

> I'm frightened of eggs, worse than frightened, they revolt me. That white round thing without any holes . . . have you ever seen anything more revolting than an egg yolk breaking and spilling its yellow liquid? Blood is jolly, red. But egg yolk is yellow, revolting. I've never tasted it.[16]

On a quite literal level, Hitchcock is lying. Patrick McGilligan notes that Hitchcock biographer John Russell Taylor stopped him mid-interview, as Hitch reported that he would end his evenings in 1917 with the Royal Engineers eating poached eggs on toast, shouting, "Aha! You said you never ate eggs!" to which Hitchcock conceded, "Well, I suppose I did eat one or two eggs when I was very young."[17] Hitchcock expresses fear and disdain for eggs, the female reproductive body, in almost textbook language that gender scholars employ to explain patriarchal fears of the feminine: the seepage and fluidity across membranes; the lack of consistent, rigid or discrete boundaries (in opposition to the clear articulation of the phallus).

These gendered associations become all the more stronger perhaps when we place his remark, "I've never tasted it," in the context of his many professions of never having sexual contact with a woman (apart from one act of procreation). The squeamishness, which became part of the canon of anecdotes about the director, may or may not be feigned. For the purposes of this argument, it is much less important to determine the veracity of Hitchcock's feelings than it is to acknowledge that his purported ovophobia became public knowledge, thanks to his promotion of the story, and that the reiteration of these feelings contributed to the public profile of a man who recoiled from the feminine.

Traces of Hitchcock's disdain for eggs can be discerned in several of his films; images of, and allusions to, eggs are often unappetizing or simply off-putting. In *To Catch a Thief*, the difficult, willful mother Jessie (Jessie Royce Landis) extinguishes a cigarette right into the yolk center of a fried egg. The gesture is an echo of an earlier image Hitchcock filmed in *Rebecca*, where another strong maternal figure Mrs. Van Hopper (Florence Bates) puts out a cigarette in a jar of white cold cream. In both scenes, the woman mars a pristine surface and thereby renders it unusable or inedible. In a Freudian vein, we may perceive the strong women as extinguishing the phallus in a fluid, amorphous (read: feminine) substance. Both women may be perceived as castrating, particularly in *Thief*. The final joke of the film bemusedly reveals that John Robie will live in a not-so-happily-after, where he will be constantly checked by the influence of Jessie, Francey's mother.

In *Under Capricorn*, the newly empowered Lady Henrietta Flusky (Ingrid Bergman) auditions three of her staff for the role of cook, proclaiming that the one who makes the best bacon, eggs, toast, and coffee would get the job. The three resulting plates are all thoroughly unappetizing, and Charles Adair (Michael Wilding) disdainfully drips the runny yolks from his fork repeatedly. In *Sabotage*, Ted Spenser (John Loder), while trying to court Mrs. Verloc (Sylvia Sidney) by pampering her and her young brother Stevie (Desmond Tester) at a nice lunch, declares, "Poached eggs, here at Simpson's? Well, it's enough to make the roast beef turn in its gravy!" Stevie responds, "He is too dignified to eat eggs," demonstrating his growing hero worship of Ted. Lastly, in *Spellbound,* psychiatrist Constance (Ingrid Bergman) jokes to her lover, "I'm glad you didn't dream about me as an eggbeater, as one of my patients did." In both *The Ring* and *To Catch a Thief,* raw eggs are thrown in a gesture of contempt.

The second bit of Hitchcock trivia that deserves contemplation in the regard of the gendered dimensions of Hitchcock's strategic shaping of public persona is his disgust with pregnant women, specifically his wife Alma, at the time of her pregnancy with Patricia. Neither biographer John Russell Taylor nor Patrick McGilligan address this subject in their books, nor does daughter Patricia in her memoir, though Donald Spoto mentions it as a tale that circulated among Hitchcock's peers. Spoto quotes an actress-friend of the director, whom he neglects to name:

> In the beginning the idea [of Alma's pregnancy] pleased him, but then as little Alma grew larger and larger with child, he began to hate her appearance. He resented her—looked on her as misshapen and ugly, and the pregnancy disgusted him.[18]

Spoto predictably casts this disgust as a product of Hitchcock's own projected self-loathing. He writes of the repulsion, "She was, after all, becoming distended, bloated—beginning, perhaps he thought, to resemble himself."[19] I am more reluctant than Spoto to attribute Hitchcock's reported disgust to narcissistic injury, though I would concede that it may have been unsettling for Hitchcock to watch his wife grow into the very shape that he had come to loathe in himself.

While this piece of biographical trivia seemed to float freely as part of Hitchcockian lore, it is certainly not a story that Hitchcock used and recycled in his many encounters with media. This discretion makes sense, particularly in deference to the feelings of his wife. Yet, the story's circulation was certainly not hindered by his remarks like "I hate pregnant women, because then they have children."[20] In this instance, Hitchcock was discussing the pregnancy of Vera Miles, which—quite solipsistically—he took to be an act of betrayal. Hitchcock had planned to mentor Miles into a movie star by featuring her as Madeleine Elster/Judy Barton in *Vertigo,* and she was forced to back out at the last minute because of her pregnancy. Thus, this resentment about pregnancy had a particular cause that was not at all rooted in his repulsion by the pregnant female form. However, the long life of the pregnancy trivia seems to have bolstered the public perception of Hitchcock's "difficulty" with women and their bodies.

Loss, danger, absence: The semiotics of Hitchcock's filmic children

Many critics have noted the relative dearth of both children and pregnant women in Hitchcock's body of work. When pregnancy does arise in a Hitchcock plot, it is often "ill-scheduled," as McGilligan points out; we see the various crises arising from unexpected pregnancies in *Rebecca, Lifeboat, Strangers on a Train* and *Marnie.*[21] In *Rebecca* and *Strangers on a Train,* we watch female villains wield a pregnancy (even if fictitious) to engage in emotional blackmail; in *Lifeboat,* a dead child becomes a mother's occasion for suicide. In *Marnie,* teenage Bernice Edgar (Louise Latham) must raise Marnie by prostituting herself after getting pregnant by a local boy who then abandons her.

Children fail to appear, even as marginal characters, in over twenty of Hitchcock's films.[22] In many of his major films—*The Lodger, The 39 Steps, Rebecca, Notorious, Dial M for Murder, Vertigo, Psycho, Frenzy*—children are absent, save for the occasional crowd or street scene. In others, children play only the smallest of roles—a child violin student in *Torn Curtain,* street hoodlums in *Mr. and Mrs. Smith,* diner customers in *Family Plot,* a hat thief in *Foreign Correspondent.* Occasionally, children may play an instrumental role in advancing the plot without having substantial speaking parts—the Boy Scout in *Stage Fright,* Betty and Hank in the two versions of *The Man Who Knew Too Much,* Jennifer's son Arnie in *The Trouble with Harry,* the bully in Hitchcock's *Blackmail* cameo (discussed at length in Chapter 3). And, of course, there is the other cameo Hitchcock filmed with a child: Hitchcock sitting in a hotel lobby in *Torn Curtain* bouncing a baby on his knee, who proceeds to wet himself.

One of the more unconventional aspects of Hitchcock's representation of children is the rarity of their appearance in the context of a wholesome, fully populated nuclear family—exceptions include the Burgoyne children in *Young and Innocent,* the Lawrence and McKenna families of *The Man Who Knew Too Much,* and the Newtons of *Shadow of a Doubt.* When children *do* appear in Hitchcock's film world, they are often immured in dangerous, unstable, or even lethal situations. In both versions of *The Man Who Knew Too Much,* the central child figure is kidnapped and held for an irregular ransom—the silence of the parents. In *Lifeboat,* a child dies in the opening scenes. *Marnie* and *Spellbound* use children in flashbacks to dramatize the primal traumas—both of them, murders—that have caused the adult leads to develop amnesia and profound neuroses. In *The Birds,* schoolchildren are menaced by bird attacks, first at Cathy Brenner's birthday party, and then as they leave their schoolhouse, and Hitchcock certainly does not spare us from witnessing the violence unleashed on their bodies.

In what has been considered the most controversial (mis)use of children in Hitchcock's cinema, *Sabotage*'s likable preteen Stevie, younger brother of Mrs. Verloc, is killed after he unwittingly carries a bomb (concealed in a film canister) onto a crowded bus. The death of the innocent child—made more sentimentally egregious by a scene just prior to the explosion in which he interacts playfully with a puppy on the bus—became the focal criticism of the film by audiences and reviewers. In later days, Hitchcock expressed regret for this turn in the plot, though he made it very clear that his regrets were attributable not to the violation of youthful innocence, but to the violation of his own formula of narrative suspense. In a 1949 essay entitled "The Enjoyment of Fear," Hitchcock chastises himself for having broken his own cardinal rule:

> Now, that episode [the bus explosion] in *Sabotage* was a direct negation of the invisible cloak of protection worn by sympathetic characters in motion pictures. In addition, because the audience knew the film can contained a bomb and the boy did not, to permit the bomb to explode was a violation of the rule forbidding a direct combination of suspense and terror.[23]

Elsewhere, he explains that the audience requires a relief from extended suspense, a sort of emotional decompressing, that *Sabotage* failed to provide in its assassination of Stevie. In the above excerpt, Hitchcock shows his awareness of the sentimental conventions that govern contemporary cinema, but he does not apologize for departing from those conventions. Instead, he frames the scenario as an aesthetic error, and thus consciously distances himself from the discourse of *pathos* that might have made him appear more vulnerable or guided by emotion.

It is reasonable to assume that Hitchcock's chosen genre—the thriller—may not inherently be conducive to the dramatization of the wholesome nuclear family and the world of children. The family signifies stability, harmony, and order, whereas the Hitchcockian thriller revels in a destabilized, often nightmarish, world of chaos and paranoia. Thus, it is not surprising that few of his films delve into the family life of middle America (*Shadow of a Doubt* excepted). Representationally, however, we must concede that, even granting this generic predisposition to focus on adulthood, children are curiously sparse in his movies. In Hitchcock's films, just as in his public appearances, children are not spared from aggression or contempt, nor do they wear the "invisible cloak of protection" that prevailing ideologies about childhood's sanctity are inclined to bestow upon them. Aggression derived from Hitchcock's own dark memories of abusive children, coupled with his self-perceived need to affirm his image as anti-maternal, anti-sentimental, create depictions of childhood that deviate meaningfully from the films of his contemporaries of classical Hollywood.

The Wrong Man and the appetites of Cain and Abel

Hitchcock's 1956 *The Wrong Man* is a great film, and a critically under-investigated one.[24] The film has several qualities that make it perhaps less legible than most in the context of the Hitchcock oeuvre. This illegibility as a Hitchcock product may explain its poor box office performance.[25] Film critic Richard Schickel refers to it as "off the main line of Hitchcock productions," and director Peter Bogdanovich celebrates it as "the kind of Hitchcock you don't expect, which is what gives it its extraordinary impact."[26] It is a departure for him in several ways. Besides the fact that it is much more consciously indebted to the film noir tradition than any of his other films, it is also his only film with nonfiction source material. Because it dramatically reenacts real life events, Hitchcock refrained from making a cameo appearance, and instead appears in silhouette before the film opens, introducing the narrative as an actuality.[27]

For the purposes of this chapter, I focus on an unusual aspect of *The Wrong Man*, which was released the same year as his much better known and more highly regarded remake of *The Man Who Knew Too Much*. Despite the film's noir leanings and its cinema vérité aesthetic, it contains undoubtedly the most idealized portrayal of a child and more specifically, of a father-son relationship, of all of his films. The father-son relationship and the fraternal rivalry that the film depicts is far from the dramatic center of the film, which focuses predominantly on the case of Manny Balestrero who has been wrongly accused of serial robbery. Consequently, the sons of Manny occupy relatively little screen time, as the film primarily unfolds to the incarceration of Manny, his further indictment through unfortunate circumstances (fueled by the ineptitude of eyewitnesses and the cruel workings of chance), and the act of grace that returns him to a (slightly diminished) family as a bastion of security and secure identity. Though the representation of the Balestrero children is peripheral to the crime story, the children's storyline functions as an important narrative and emotional counterpoint to the dramatically hefty tale of persecution and unpalatable injustice. In addition, the exploration of father-son and brotherly dynamics presents an unprecedented set of dramatic opportunities through which Hitchcock may have dealt with his ambivalences toward childhood, masculinity, and paternal acceptance.

Sibling rivalry very rarely appears in Hitchcock's body of work. Brothers and sisters may bicker (*Young and Innocent, Shadow of a Doubt, Strangers on a Train*), but their contest of wills almost never takes center stage.[28] One exception is an episode of *The Alfred Hitchcock Hour*, entitled "The Crimson Witness," in which a man loses his job, his wife, and mistress to an overachieving brother, and decides to murder him. Because of Hitchcock's reluctance to speak about his family, it is difficult to understand the intricacies of the relationship he had with his own siblings. As mentioned, he was born seven and nine years after his sister and brother, and he had very little contact with them, particularly after leaving England for America. Older brother William, whom Spoto describes as "large and barrel-chested and awkward," and a cousin described as "well-built," served as Hitchcock's best man at his wedding, though they visited each other very little afterwards.[29]

According to reports from those close to the family, Hitchcock resented his brother, whom he dismissed as a user, claiming William would only visit to drink their wine. Playwright Charles Bennett recalled that Hitchcock disdainfully pronounced his brother, "large, prosperous, and dull." William, Jr. *was*, in fact, prosperous; after taking control of his father's business upon his death, he sold the grocery at a great profit to a larger market conglomerate. While Hitchcock's remarks about his brother are spare, they may be instructive as to the nature of their relationship. Hitchcock felt he had perhaps disappointed his father by refusing to cast his lot with the family business, and therefore, William may have generated a degree of envy in him. Moreover, the masculinity of the "well-built," "barrel-chested" brother was quite the antithesis of his own "cottage-loaf" shaped body, resembling his mother's.

In *The Wrong Man*, protagonist Manny (Henry Fonda) is a working-class jazz musician from Long Island who plays at an upscale club in New York City to make ends meet for his young wife Rose (Vera Miles), and their two sons, Bob, 8, (Kippy Campbell), and Greg, 5 (Robert Essen). After Manny is mistakenly identified—by several easily influenced witnesses—as the perpetrator of a series of robberies, the film depicts his incarceration and search to clear his name, and equally importantly, it depicts the great emotional damage inflicted on the family as they stand by Manny, and are repeatedly let down by the justice system. Rose undergoes a nervous breakdown, from which she cannot recover by the film's end, though an insert at the film's close informs the audience that the family is well, and residing in Florida. The film is darker, with a greater sense of seriousness and melancholy than most of his other films from the 1950s apart from *Vertigo*.

The young brothers Bob and Greg occupy a small amount of screen time, though Hitchcock takes care in portraying them as distinct from one another in their temperaments and behaviors. The film introduces them early, as Bob tattles on younger Greg for playing the "mouth organ" while Bob is practicing the piano. Manny joins the two boys in the living room to referee. He praises Bob for his musical potential and encourages Greg, expressing confidence that he was coming to understand the melody. Hitchcock's physical framing of the scene, however, shows us Manny's inclination toward the older child. Greg remains alone in the far left of the frame, as Manny seats himself beside his older son, clutching and patting his arm, in the far right. Thus, the camera gives us a visual understanding of the siblings' dynamics with the father that may belie his seeming neutrality. Manny promises his two sons that he will give them music lessons that evening, fifteen minutes each, when Greg interrupts with, "Me first!"

Just before Manny is arrested and fails to return home as usual, the police call the Balestrero household. As the phone rings, we see young Greg in the foreground with his mother, as he hovers, watching her cut a pie crust in the kitchen. In the background, Bob answers the phone, responding that his father would be home at 5:30 p.m. The framing here of Greg with his mother in the kitchen suggests their closeness, recalling a younger Hitchcock whose most intense childhood bond was with his mother, and who spent a great deal of time in the kitchen with her.

The scene that most effectively differentiates the two boys is that of Manny's first homecoming from jail. Bob cries out, "Dad!" and runs into the arms of his father, leaving Greg off to the side, to cling at his coat. In the following scene, Bob enters his father's bedroom, where Manny is reclining on the bed. Almost immediately, Bob expresses his reluctance to hear any allegations against his father, protesting, "Dad, you're the best dad in the world!" Clearly moved, Manny responds, "I hope you never have to go through what I went through, and if you do, I hope you have a son just like mine to come back to." Throughout the scene, father and son exchange words in a shot-reverse shot sequence, framing them each in a medium close-up, conveying a sense of intimacy often reserved for scenes of love and seduction. As Manny dramatically muses, "I never knew what my boys meant to me until right now," Bob cries out, and they embrace in a tight two-shot. As they disengage from the hug, the camera remains in a two-shot, even as they begin to separate.

In the final shot of the scene, father and son clasp hands tightly, as Bob usurps the paternal rôle and advises his father, "You'd better get some sleep." The close focus on the hands is important, as there are several close-ups on Manny's hands at key moments in the film—as he strums his double bass at the Stork Club, as he examines his clenched fists in the jail cell (displaying anger, fear, and a sense of revoked agency), and later, as he tousles his wife Rose's hair in an effort to revive her spirit. Bob, then, is linked to this hand motif, perhaps even further because, like his father, he uses his hands to play a musical instrument (as opposed to younger, "mouthier" Greg, who plays the harmonica). This father-son exchange is without a doubt the most sentimental, emotionally expressive scene between a father and child in all of Hitchcock's work.

The film cuts abruptly from the father-son embrace to the kitchen table, in a medium shot of young Greg shoveling fork after fork of lasagna into his mouth. The tone is so markedly different; the transition almost registers as comic. We have been transported without warning from the clasping masculine hands, to the gaping, overflowing mouth of the ravenous child. Framed inches from Greg's head, and at the same level, is a cookie jar, and a tall half-drunk glass of milk sits before him. Twice in the film, when Manny returns home from work, he picks up two quarts of milk sitting on the stoop (suggesting his arrival home in the early morning), before entering the house and checking in on his sleeping children first, then Rose. Manny is established from the outset as a good provider, and here in this kitchen scene, Greg is positioned as the consumer—the boy who is much more interested in lasagna and milk than the fate of his father in the eyes of the law.[30] Later, when Greg complains that their father has failed in his promise to give them music lessons, Bob dutifully points out the larger problems that surround Manny. In the film's final shot, as the Balestrero family walks arm in arm down a Florida avenue lined with palm trees, we can see, even in extreme long shot, that Manny embraces Bob, as Rose holds Greg close.

The above characterizations are subtleties that certainly have little influence over the film's narrative arc, though it is interesting to note the nuances of character, particularly in the two sons, that resonate with Hitchcock's own childhood experience. Like the younger sibling Greg, he was a heavy eater, partial to his mother, and ultimately more remote from his father. His possible identification with the younger child may have been an expression of guilt—the kind Hitchcock demonstrated in speaking of the "disappointment" his father felt toward him. It is important to realize, however, that Greg's behavior was in part the result of his age—most five-year-old boys are developmentally quite far behind eight-year-olds, and less capable of the empathy Bob demonstrates. What is more, Bob's position as the favored child of the father may not in fact be a privileged one.

David Sterritt, in his critique of *The Wrong Man*, reasons that Manny, as a product of the cowardly conformist and conservative culture of 1950s America, is perhaps the "wrong man" in the crime for which he was charged, but is not at all free from guilt. According to Sterritt, Manny is guilty "of failing to surmount his submissive impulses, of failing to overcome a deep malaise that informs his life, of failing to avoid a perception of decay in the middle-class."[31] Thus, Greg's decision to indulge in lasagna and sidestep the bathetic melodrama of the class oppression responsible for the family's struggles may, in the world of 1950s New York, be as good as any. Certainly Hitchcock distrusted, and wanted no part of, this class melodrama. Therefore, we may read an unresolved ambivalence into the film, in terms of paternal identification. If Hitchcock used the dramatic milieu of the Balestrero household to explore the various alignments and allegiances between parents and children, he may have expressed both a sense of disappointment and relief surrounding his failed paternal identification and communion.

It should be clear from the above discussion of children in and outside the director's work that Hitchcock carefully tailored his perceived relationship to children, and in doing so, papered the cracks of a troubled relation to his own past. Through the performance of his ironized relation to youth, he hoped to forestall and possibly negate any fast and easy connections among the often connotatively linked tropes of fatness, sentimentality, and effeminacy. Many actors report, in fact, that Hitchcock enjoyed warm relations with most children. According to actress Anna Lee, he "was nicer to children than he was to adults." Veronica Cartwright, who played young Cathy Brenner in *The Birds*, recalls, "I had heard that Hitchcock didn't like kids. It was just a rumor, and I must say that he was always very nice and kind with me."[32]

This disconnect between actuality and manicured reputation is perhaps analogous to the disparity between the descriptions Hitchcock would offer of his literary tastes and cinematic influences (Griffith, Galsworthy, Shaw, Buchan, Bennett—all men), and the creative writing environment in which he actually worked, which never lacked women (Alma, Joan Harrison, Marie Belloc Lowndes, Ethel Lina White). In fact, 32 (24 percent) of Hitchcock's 122 writers were women—not at all an insignificant portion. In a 1935 interview, Hitchcock vowed, "I shall continue to keep the atmosphere of my films largely masculine."[33] It is a rather curious phrasing, and perhaps impenetrable, but whatever may constitute a "masculine environment," neither Hitchcock's diegetic worlds nor his creative enclaves were ever without strong feminine influence. Hitchcock's public disavowals of the feminine and the young were, in many contexts, disingenuous, and they were certainly indicative of an artist who felt quite vulnerable regarding how his body was read by the public, and who felt the need to redraw the often smudged lines of masculinity that defined his legendary image.

6

Hitchcock and the queer lens of fatness

The previous chapter demonstrated that Hitchcock's flamboyant anti-child stance, articulated in his public persona and in his representational strategies of children in film, may signify a strong desire to be read as conforming to the mandates of conventional heterosexual masculinity, in an attempt to divorce himself from the cultural paradigm that links fatness with femininity and maternity. In trying to shape his reputation as resolutely unsentimental and resistant to nurturing roles, he aligned himself curiously with conservatively gendered rhetorical positions. Paradoxically, his refusal to enshrine the child figure as the sentimental and semiotic center of affective relations and as the linchpin of the heterosexual nuclear family carries strong queer reverberations as well.

Lee Edelman has described the conventional, politically bipartisan pro-child stance as encompassing and promoting a worldview that entails the consummation of adult heterosexual monogamy and procreation as the desired end of social relations and the guarantor of the cultural reproduction of sameness over time, which generates the illusory marriage of identity to futurity, and thus forges a compelling, if imagined, stability of the coherent reproductive subject.[1] Hitchcock's refusal to acknowledge the premium status of the child as guarantor of identity, then, registers as queer critique. In other words, we may interpret Hitchcock's anti-child rhetoric as embracing heteronormativity through conventional gender performance, yet critiquing it through the refusal of the figure around which traditional heterosexuality coalesces.

This final chapter takes an opportunity to explore Hitchcock from a new perspective, grounded in the overlapping discourses of fat studies and queer theory. It argues that Hitchcock's removal from the dominant paradigms of patriarchal love and romance endowed him with a critical view of conventional heterosexuality and a savvy and innovatively queer understanding of the complexity of cinematic desire and identification. By acknowledging the abject qualities of his own body, which signified disorder, lack of discipline, the exceeding of proper and normal corporeal boundaries, he saw that the binaries in place that valorized and abjected different bodies, relationships, and feelings were quite tenuously upheld, and that great drama could emerge from engaging the radical disparity between appearance and reality vis-à-vis the "normal" and "stable" body, and the putatively "healthy" relationship.

Before examining Hitchcock's cinema, and his filmmaking practices, it is important to understand the various disciplinary and political affinities between fat studies and queer theory, as well as how they have fed one another through paradigms of resistance and critique. Fat studies and queer theory (and by extension LGBTQ studies) are organized around marginalized bodies and identities. They are both activist-based movements, and have histories that date back at least thirty years (longer for LGBT activism). According to Marilyn Wann, "The fat pride community, often called the size acceptance movement, began in the United States with the National Association to Advance Fat Acceptance in 1969 and the powerful work of the Fat Underground in the 1970s."[2] The timing is significant here; while earlier forms of organizing within the queer community had preceded the above projects by twenty years or so—the Daughters of Bilitis, the Mattachine Society, and homophile movement—1969 is, of course, the watershed LGBTQ moment in the eruption of violence at the Stonewall Inn, and its legendary aftermath. For both movements, the 1970s became a time of nascent wide-scale organizing, though queer visibility perhaps surpassed that of the Fat Underground.

Both movements took aim at social and economic policies, national and state legislation, and public environments that fostered discrimination against bodies perceived as pathological or undeserving of the rights and privileges reserved for the normative citizen. In the intervening years queer politics has taken up the fights of immigration, gay marriage, adoption, fostering, job discrimination, recognition and research for the AIDS epidemic, hate crime legislation, domestic privacy, the right to practice as doctors and work as educators, and countless other avenues seeking equality, protection, and respect. Weight and size acceptance activists faced similar and contiguous challenges. They also fought to expose job discrimination, social discrimination (particularly in schools), pathologization and neglect in the medical community, limitations on adoption, class-based ideologies that simultaneously implicate the fat and the poor, oppressive standards of beauty and health manufactured by the fashion industry, clothing designers, advertisers, pageant culture, and broader orchestrations of popular culture.

In his exploration of twentieth-century fat masculinity in America in *Fat Boys*, Sander Gilman addresses the question of normativity, as it is exercised regarding bodies of size and their gender. For him, the questions "of what fat is and what a man is, assume the existence of a 'normal' ideal of both weight and masculinity." He posits the construction of the "reasonable man" in legal discourse, *from* whom we imagine acceptable behavior and social obligation, and *for* whom rights are guaranteed. And thus, he finds that

> while the reasonable man is merely an imaginary character, the various descriptions and embellishments by the judiciary and the commentators attribute to him characteristics and personality traits that in turn can be used to further flesh out the identity of the reasonable man. His body cannot be that of a fat man; rather, it is the archetypal body that defines the normal male.[3]

The presumed subject of judicial and legislative discourse, then, is not only presumed (heterosexual) male, but also one of normative size. By extension, then, the "reasonable" subject is linked to masculinity and moderation in size and appetites. Both the fat and queer body fall outside of acceptable measures of citizenship. The cultural hierarchies of bodies—the procreative over the non-procreative; the efficient, disciplined body over the inefficient, superfluous body; the healthy body over the ill body—displace both subjects, often using the same rationales. And of course, the language of death—"morbid" obesity and the association of gayness with AIDS—looms within the signifying regime that describes, and inscribes, both groups.

When it comes to mass culture and popular entertainment, negative and absent representation has been a shared struggle by both fat and queer communities. Representations of LGBT characters in film and television have historically tended to be monstrous, villainous, deserving of contempt or pity, or a source of ridicule or humor. Fat representation has certain similarities to queer signification in terms of its position in the entertainment world; the fat person functions as the butt of jokes, as visual spectacle, or as a figure of pity, plagued by loneliness, regret, and social ostracism. There is, to be sure, a certain overlap in the historical reception of fat and queer characters, just as there has been in terms of fat and queer cultural reception at large: the evocation of disgust. The notion of disgust as a physical, visceral bodily reaction has further complicated both fat and queer politics.

The idea that queer sex practices or the mere visibility of excess fat on the body may produce a nausea or revulsion in the phobic spectator/citizen seems to give credence to a kind of empirical proof that the offended subjects are responding to the presence of something "unnatural," which can be felt by the body. This dangerous elision of culturally produced affect with essentialist body response has been wielded by anti-fat and anti-gay (and particularly anti-trans) contingencies as evidence of the "unnatural" status of queer and fat bodies. The fact that even bodily processes (particularly peristalsis, the mechanism by which we swallow and vomit) are mental ones as well, and that ideological conditioning may be responsible for training and producing these "natural" responses of revulsion, is overlooked in these simplistic accounts of disgust as a "natural warning" against unhealthy or dangerous otherness.

The unsophisticated understanding of the relationships among bodies, ideologies, and affect and the tendency to misconstrue the mechanism of physical disgust have hindered progress by fat and queer activists. Another obstacle faced by activists of both contingencies is the persistent and seemingly indelible misapprehension of the fat body and the queer body as products of conscious choice. The notion that one chooses to be gay or fat attenuates the very grounds on which activists stand, in terms of their being stymied by a public perception of their organizing around a matter that they could eradicate or control themselves, had they any sense of discipline, morality, or conscience.

Whereas activism based in race and gender may have a certain perceived claim to authenticity or a marginalization rooted in bodily "truth," the gay and fat subject are often falsely understood to have made their own bed, even more so because both subjects are defined by their "vices" of gluttony and perversion. These insufficient understandings of queerness and fatness derive from the perception of sexuality as an act of will, and body size as a simple product of the economy of diet and exercise that should be followed. The genetic bases of orientation and body composition remain uninvestigated and unreferenced, as they complicate the story of identity acquisition, and thus become inconvenient, and therefore jettisoned, as extraneous or insignificant factors in determining the makeup of the subject. Regarding both the fat and the queer body, the prevailing normative sentiment is that the marginalized subject simply *isn't trying hard enough* to conform or self-correct.

Hitchcock certainly experienced his body as non-normative, and I do not imply here that because Hitchcock's body did not conform to normative standards of acceptable masculinity, he came to discount the "truth" or validity of normative standards wholesale. In fact, he perceived his fatness as a failing, a falling short, and his yardstick clearly marked the measurements of ingrained normativity. Yet, I believe that one may feel acutely the narcissistic injury of social exclusion and at the same time critique the assumptions underlying normativity, without the critique necessarily originating from a "sour grapes" mentality. And this chapter argues that Hitchcock's investment in the proper body was also counterweighted by deep suspicions of the normative's fictive, artificial, and coercive properties.

In this regard, I argue for the importance of looking at Hitchcock's own queerness, registered by both his body and his sensitivity to the fictions of hegemony. To argue for Hitchcock's queerness is not to suggest that he was a homosexual, either in his sexual practices or in his private self-perception, nor is it to exonerate him from allegations of homophobia and misogyny on many fronts. Hitchcock, of course, chose a life of heterosexual monogamy and procreation, though he portrays himself time and again as conforming to the letter of patriarchal law, but not necessarily its spirit. Understanding the queer nature of Hitchcock and his cinema in particular importantly exempts him from being treated with formulaic accounts of cinematic processes of desire and identification that traditionally have underwritten the agenda of what Lee Edelman has called the "absolute value of reproductive futurism."[4]

Hitchcock and the fat closet

Eve Kosofsky Sedgwick and Michael Moon, in their playfully ambitious, multiform essay, "Divinity: A Dossier, A Performance Piece, A Little-Understood Emotion," approach the social construction of the gay closet as one that may have a ready corollary in the world of fat women—a fat closet. Michael Moon describes this closet in terms of its affinities with the closet of homosexual identity, in its issues of (non)secrecy, social intelligibility, and the distribution of knowledge about the fat subject. He writes:

> The closet seems to function as a closet to the degree that it's a glass closet, the secret to the degree that it's an open one. . . . Incredibly, in this society everyone who sees a fat woman feels they know something about her that she doesn't herself know. . . . [Spectators of the fat woman feel as if they have] a privileged narrative understanding of her will (she's addicted), her history (she's frustrated), her perception (she can't see herself as she really looks), her prognosis (she's killing herself).[5]

In this passage, Moon maps fat self-awareness, and others' awareness of a woman's fatness, onto the model of the open homosexual secret—a facet of one's identity that is discursively constrained through the taboo of its utterance, though simultaneously a figure of obvious and (through its obviousness) degrading signification. Though Moon and Sedgwick establish the parallelism of the fat and gay closets as specifically pertinent to the fat woman, the same semiotic register applies in the case of the fat man. Sander Gilman echoes Moon's sentiment about the open secret, applying it to the contemporary fat male, when he writes, "Fat men's bodies seem to be 'readable' to everyone but fat men themselves."[6] Gilman's observation rests on an unspoken assumption that if the fat subject, male or female, truly *knew* of their fatness, they would do something about it. As it stands, then, fatness reads as both social abjection and profound lack of self-awareness.

Sedgwick then takes her cue from Moon's description of the fat closet, remarking on the impact of rhetorical disclosure in the form of fat confession—an analog, of course, to the act of "coming out" as gay.

> It follows from all this, however, that there is such a process as coming out as a fat woman. . . . It involves the risk of uttering bathetically as a brave declaration that truth which can scarcely in this instance ever have been less than self-evident. Coming out for a fat woman . . . is a way of staking one's claim to insist on, and participate actively in, a renegotiation of the representational contract between one's body and one's world.

Again, Sedgwick theorizes the fat female positionality and its relation to this disclosure, but I would argue that the same kind of "risk" is at stake in male confession, even if there are markedly different, gendered reception processes (due to women's vulnerability in making proclamations about their body, their status as visual spectacle, the "presumptuousness" of a woman narrating her own body, etc.).

This queer notion of the fat closet and the act of "coming out" as fat has particular resonance with Hitchcock as a cultural icon and filmmaker. In certain ways, Hitchcock, with his never-ending supply of fat jokes, may be seen to have preemptively smashed any "closet" of marginalization to bits. And certainly, preemption must have been one of Hitchcock's major motives for staking territory as the first, and therefore only, one to make comment on his weight and size. His profound desire to be in control over the public's perception of him made it crucial that he not be read as not "in" on the joke of his fatness. Secondly, to declare his fatness was to forestall anyone else's declaration of it. Obviously, this was not true with the press (as we see throughout Chapter 1), who took every chance to refer to the weight and the girth of the director. But Hitchcock's self-confession of fatness seemed to foreclose the mention of it in his presence.

Thus, while he may have taken every opportunity to dispel doubts about his self-awareness by reminding the world that he was in on the fat joke, the closet persisted in the casting of his size (in his personal and professional life) as an "open secret." This strange manifestation of closeted fatness perhaps has its greatest illustration in the anecdote of Tippi Hedren's verbal tussle with Hitchcock on the set of *Marnie*. When the director declined to give Hedren a weekend off from shooting to go to New York City to accept an award for *Photoplay* magazine's Star of Tomorrow, she flew into a rage, reportedly calling him a "fat pig." This confrontation all but severed their working relationship and certainly capsized their already shaky personal relationship.[7] Hitchcock later described the event to his biographer John Russell Taylor. "She did what no one is permitted to do. She referred to my weight."[8]

It is difficult to know if Hitchcock's indignation at this slight was at all ironic or if it was simply one of hurt and anger. Either way, the notion of the "open secret" as something taboo in its articulation becomes quite evident. Hitchcock's weight—something that everyone knew, but no one spoke of except him—parallels the subject of homosexuality in the making of his 1948 film *Rope*. Screenwriter Arthur Laurents, in an interview, shares the following:

> What was curious to me was—*Rope* is obviously about homosexuals. The word was never mentioned. Not by Hitch. Not by anybody at Warners where it was filmed. It was referred to as *It*. They were going to do a picture about *It*. And the actors were *It*.[9]

Laurents further suggests that the film performed much better in Europe than it did in the States because its people were more comfortable with *It*. Just as same-sex desire was the great unnameable in the process of creating the film, Hitchcock's weight was unnameable, save by the director himself. Both instances of censorship hinge on the naming of a marginal or socially degraded position. Thus, like the LGBT subject, Hitchcock was acutely aware of the constant potential to be hurt or embarrassed through assaultive language of his body's social unacceptability.

It may seem curious or counterintuitive that the director may have insulted himself in public, unabashedly and often, while he remained intimidated and bothered by the threat of humiliation by a familiar's use of the same language. In her 1997 *Excitable Speech*, Judith Butler's discussion of hate speech, interpellation, and performativity provides some welcome enlightenment on the subject of the qualitative differences between the self-implicating utterance and the accusation from the other. While "hate speech" may be a seemingly ridiculous way to characterize casual fat jokes or observations, the language of fatness used against an intended audience references a host of cultural connotations that loom much larger than the immediate rhetorical situation of the joke or comment.

To call someone "fat" is to evoke a signifying chain of injurious ideas, which have been put in the service of creating fat-phobic and fat-hating publics. To be called by these words is to experience a violent interpellation; one is called into their subjectivity in these instances by a naming which links their public recognition with their social stigma.[10] One's choice to apply the language of fatness oneself constitutes an act of interpellation, to be sure, but one over which the speaker has control (mechanical control, if not semiotic). Thus, while Hitchcock's naming his fatness may perform the rhetorical work of Sedgwick's description—"insist[ing] on, and participat[ing] actively in, a renegotiation of the representational contract between one's body and one's world," hearing the words from another, whether a friendly intimate or a hostile employee (like Hedren), may constitute a traumatizing ontological confrontation.[11] The language of queerness is similar in its very different qualitative value depending on who is employing it.

A sense of sex: Queer romance in Hitchcock's cinema

> Repressed sex is more constructive for the creative person. It must get out, and so it goes into the work. I think it helped create a sense of sex in my work.[12]

Hitchcock is right; we may find many "senses of sex" in his work. And both the senses and the sensibilities of the sex in his films are very often queer. He portrayed rather few overtly LGBT characters in his body of work: Mrs. Danvers in *Rebecca*; Isobel Sedbusk and companion in *Suspicion*; Philip and Brandon in *Rope*; Bruno Anthony in *Strangers on a Train*; Leonard in *North by Northwest*.[13] There are many more, though, who read as queer on more subtle registers of performance and sign: Handel Fane in *Murder!*; The General in *Secret Agent*; Uncle Charlie in *Shadow of a Doubt*; Andre LaTour in *The Paradine Case*; Commodore Gill in *Stage Fright*; Norman Bates in *Psycho*; the titular *Marnie*; Bob Rusk in *Frenzy*, for example.

At the level of narrative and characterization, however, Hitchcock's films did not read queer through the expressed sexualities of those who populate his films as often as they did through the persistent, sometimes merciless, critique of conventional heterosexual romance contained so often therein. In her pioneer essay "Queer and Now," Eve Sedgwick provides a very useful definition of queer, insofar as the term may point to moments and places when and where "the constituent elements of anyone's gender, of anyone's sexuality aren't made (or *can't* be made) to signify monolithically."[14] The heteronormative, she argues, requires a tight and carefully policed alignment of a subject's gender identification, her gender preference, procreative choice, preferred sexual acts, sexual fantasies, main locus of emotional bonds, enjoyment of power in sexual relations, and community of cultural and political identification.[15] Queerness, then, resides in the places where this alignment fails, shifts, or proves illusory.

As discussed earlier, Hitchcock led a celibate life. His marriage to Alma was comfortably (by most accounts) companionate and housed an inspired and very successful collaboration on cinematic projects. Yet, passion was notably missing from their arrangement. It is difficult to know if their absence of physicality had more to do with an absence of physical attraction or with the impotence resulting from Hitchcock's weight and drinking (and perhaps anxiety). The fact that marriage did not compel or facilitate other forms of intimacy for him perhaps instilled in him his disillusionment about the difficulty, if not impossibility, of finding convergence of romantic love, sexual desire, platonic fulfillment, and compliance with the social contract of marriage in its various limitations and definitions. As a result of this disillusionment, Hitchcock had a degree of contempt for films that insisted on the fantasmatic easy alignments of heteronormative romance, and he perennially treated romantic love as alternately dangerous, rooted in deceit or betrayal, unstable, conditional, and as a failure of the imagination. Romantic heterosexuality in his cinema is always of suspect origin, motivation, and shelf life. Marriage, in particular, takes a hit throughout his body of work. Quite often, a spouse is a liability (*Torn Curtain*), a stifler of energies (*Rear Window*), a redundancy (*Frenzy*), a bad habit (*Mr. and Mrs. Smith*), or even a prisoner (*Marnie*).

To be fair, love is often a tremendous source of visual and narrative pleasure in the films of Hitchcock. It is certainly no sentence of existential anguish across the board. Yet, there is often a subtle undercutting of the primacy of the romantic couple's bond, sometimes as a cosmetic slight and other times as a lethal dissection of illusion-plagued dysfunction. What follows is a partial catalog of Hitchcock's portrayals of love and marriage that contain potentially queer strands of resistance and/or seeds of destruction:

1. *Love as a Trap or a Loss of Freedom*

The handcuffs of *The 39 Steps* (which Hitchcock famously used on his starring couple in an epic practical joke) physically encapsulate some of the more ambivalent feelings that Hitchcock reveals about love in his films. The handcuffs suggest the bonds of love, ideological bonds, the surrender of agency, the disappearance of freewill or solitude. The final scene, when Hannay (Robert Donat) and Pamela (Madeleine Carroll) join hands, for the first time, of their own volition, may be read optimistically as a contrasting sign of their agency as they enter into romance, or cynically that their union is yet another variation on the bondage described above. As discussed earlier, *Blackmail* similarly tropes on love as an imprisonment, as Alice finds herself "saved" by Frank, at the price of her autonomy. In *Rear Window*, Jeffries envisions marriage as the death of bachelorhood and subsequently, of freedom. When Stella remarks of Miss Lonelyhearts, "Poor soul. Maybe one day she'll find her happiness," Jeff retorts, "Yeah, and some man will lose his." While Jeff appears to have learned his lesson by the film's end, that marriage does not mean the end of freedom, we have to read this against his symbolic double castration, as he naps next to Lisa, who now literally wears the pants in the relationship. *Marnie*'s portrayal of love is the most cynical, and the most explicit in its depiction of love as both sickness and trap, which is evident in Mark's barbaric diatribe, "I've tracked you and caught you, and by god, I'm going to keep you."

2. *Love as Safety or Social Legitimacy*

Sometimes love in Hitchcock's film is firmly grounded in gratitude or appreciation of a relationship's stability or affording of privilege, but at the price of passion or intensity of desire. A kind of restlessness and shaky complacency mar the relationships of the Lawrences and the McKennas in the two versions of *The Man Who Knew Too Much*. Particularly for the wives, marriage is a site of compromise and frustration. Jill's (Edna Best) romantic attentions have strayed, and Jo (Doris Day) resents surrendering her life as a performer and yielding to her husband's wishes for no further children. The kidnappings in both films function not simply as a mechanism to execute the film's MacGuffin, but as a narrative means of reaffirming the couples' gratitude for their safety and stability, if not their passion or freewill. Guy Haines (Farley Granger) of *Strangers on a Train* faces the threat of social abjection, through the machinations of first wife Miriam (Laura Elliott), and the double threat, embodied by Bruno Anthony (Robert Walker), of implication in murder and of homoerotic interpellation, and his wife-to-be, the rather bland Anne Morton (Ruth Roman), possesses relative virtues of promising upward mobility and reassurance of his sexual identity. The relationship, however reads as quite sterile, and serves to color the superficially unimpeachable Guy with darker shades of opportunism. *The Paradine Case* and *Topaz* both dramatize the predicament of a protagonist who is caught between the seductive and potentially dangerous passions of an enigmatic woman and the relatively unglamorous domesticity embodied by their wives. While Tony Keane (Gregory Peck) returns to the safety of his loyal wife, Andre Devereaux (Frederick Stafford) loses his as a result of the affair, and at the film's end, he remains alone.

3. *Love as the Eroticization of Inequality*
Hitchcockian love is at times characterized by an attraction that forms in the midst of, or even perhaps because of, an imbalance in power or knowledge. This imbalance is, of course, a classical Hollywood paradigm of romance, and thus certainly not unique to Hitchcock, though it seems worth illuminating as a potentially queer, disruptive facet of the portrayal of romantic desire. *Spellbound* abounds with the language of the doctor and patient, of transference and countertransference, and it is incorporated playfully into the courtship rituals of blossoming couple, amnesiac John Ballantyne (Gregory Peck) and psychoanalyst Constance Petersen (Ingrid Bergman). John enters into the whirlwind romance with a fragmented, incomplete, and almost totally self-effaced memory. Constance welcomes the challenge of retrieving John's identity and winning over his trust and loyalty, thereby blurring the lines of the personal and the professional. More than in many Hitchcock films, the romance become somewhat naturalized and de-pathologized through the recovery of John's memory, and his relief that Constance fits into the profile of his prior life (single, available, ostensibly heterosexual). Yet the roots of the relationship lay visibly in the power-saturated relationship of amorous therapist and disoriented analysand. In *Lifeboat*, the central romance—to the degree that there is one—grows between the wealthy devil-may-care Constance Porter (played by Tallulah Bankhead; another Hitchcock "Constance" whose virtuous name may not fit the woman snugly) and working-class John Kovac (John Hodiak). Their near-death experiences together seem to collude in breaking down their stubbornness to realize true affection, though the attraction remains rooted in a somewhat mutually fetishistic relation between the rugged "noble savage" and the decadent "rich bitch." *Marnie,* of course, stands again as exemplary model of heterosexual critique, particularly in this optic, where the smug Mark lords his knowledge of Marnie's criminal past over her, blackmailing her into marriage against her will. In addition to this extortion, Marnie penetratingly captures the pathological doctor-patient relationship that has attached itself to the other power dynamic of hunter and prey, when she growls, "You Freud, Me Jane?" The line is a lovely, self-aware condensation of the tropes of the barbaric hunter and patriarchal the/rapist.

4. *Love Under False Pretenses*
Hitchcock intimates that all relationships are games of a sort, and that we all perform roles to our best advantage. His often used trope of theatricality (*Murder!*, *Stage Fright*, *Rear Window*) extends to the theater of heterosexual romance as well. Often a couple in a Hitchcock film begins their romance with false ideas about the identity and motives of the other. The erotic relationship

in *North by Northwest* between Roger Thornhill (Cary Grant) and Eve Kendall (Eva Marie Saint) is bolstered by the is-she-or-isn't-she intrigue generated by Eve's duplicity (resonant of biblical Eve). Here Hitchcock eroticizes the potential danger of her traitor status. In *Spellbound*, as discussed, John Ballantyne tries to pass as Dr. Edwardes to cover his amnesia, and thus his relationship with Constance begins with his mistaken identity. Johnnie Aysgarth (Cary Grant) falsely presents himself to Lina McLaidlaw (Joan Fontaine) as an eligible, wealthy, upright bachelor (*Suspicion*), much as Maxim (Laurence Olivier) introduces himself to "I" (also Fontaine) a year earlier in *Rebecca*, masking a dark and turbulent past with his first wife. In both stories, Fontaine experiences a rude awakening that causes her to re-evaluate the very foundations of her love. On a lighter, more superficial level, *The Birds* begins with Melanie Daniels's (Tippi Hedren) assumption of a false identity—that of a pet store worker—only to be one-upped by the equally duplicitous Mitch Brenner (Rod Taylor); the collision of deceit does not bode well for the couple.

5. *Love as Endangerment to Person and Personhood*

Other views of heterosexual romantic love are explored in Hitchcock's film worlds, such as their tendency to imperil one's body as well as one's sense of self. The dangerously dark and cynical view of marriage espoused by Uncle Charlie (Joseph Cotten) in *Shadow of a Doubt* casts women as parasitic heifers and men as unwitting victims who are spiritually and financially leeched by them. In both *Notorious* and *Under Capricorn*, Ingrid Bergman plays a role in which she sacrifices her virtue and suffers as a result of her need to prove her love. In both films, she whores herself to comply with what she incorrectly believes are the wishes of her lover. In *Suspicion*, Lina's opening herself to love means becoming vulnerable to the charms of a usurer and possible killer. In *The Paradine Case*, Tony Keane sacrifices the trust of his loving wife and his reputation as an upstanding barrister, all because of the distortions wrought by the sick seductions of Maddalena Paradine, played by Alida Valli, (again the name, an Italian version of Magdalene, is significant to the character). *Vertigo*, which artfully deconstructs the boundaries between romantic love and unhealthy obsession, depicts a degraded state of love that renders both subject and object incoherent and devastated.

6. *Love as Unhealthy Iteration of the Primary Oedipal Bond*

   Psycho. The Birds. Enough said.

As the above examples suggest, Hitchcock's views on heterosexual romance were complicated, and not without the recognition of their pleasures and virtues, experienced by his characters and his audiences. Yet, immanent in his portrayals of conventional love are the intimations, some subtle, some writ large, that such a love cannot succeed or maintain itself, save as a dangerous illusion. We have seen the ways in which Hitchcock has engaged these critiques of heterosexual love through representational strategies. What remains is an examination of the profound ways that Hitchcock's bodily otherness afforded an ingeniously queer perspective on the physical and psychic dimensions of spectatorship.

As a man who was deeply frustrated with his body and his romantic life, Hitchcock cherished the very mechanisms of desire and identification that transported the spectator to a pleasurable state of *having* and *being*, however illusory. It would be erroneous to assume, just because Hitchcock displayed an innately thorough knowledge of the illusion and artifice behind cinema's transformative powers, that he was immune to the pleasures of vicarious cinematic experience. To his mind, the stimuli may be artificial, but the responses were certainly not. The remainder of this chapter investigates Hitchcock's investment in processes of desire and identification, particularly as processes that are queer in their very refusal of a monolithic alignment of a presumed heterosexual subject and spectator.

There is a moment in the 2012 Hitchcock biopic *The Girl*, where Hitchcock, very drunk and inconsolably lovelorn (for Tippi Hedren), accepts a ride home from the young, handsome, and virile producer Jim Brown. With an uncharacteristic lack of self-consciousness brought on by inebriation, Hitchcock has just shared with Brown very intimate details of his sexual history: "I've never had sex with anybody else. People don't believe me. They think I say it to shock. It's true. . . . Years ago, of course. Can't get it up now. Impotent . . ." As they arrive and Brown pulls Hitchcock from the compact car, Hitch rests his arm around Brown's broad shoulders, looks him in the eye, their faces just inches apart, and vows, "I'd give it all up, Jim, the money, the films, everything I've ever done . . ." "No girl is worth that," Brown interrupts compassionately. But Hitchcock continues: ". . . to be like you. To look like you." Thanks to Toby Jones's layered portrayal of him, the moment is complicated. As Hitchcock gazes at what he considers to be an ideal male specimen (or, at least, a sexually viable one), we can read wistfulness, sincerity, tenderness, perhaps a hint of antagonism, and undeniable attraction.

In a film largely devoted to depicting Hitchcock as an unhappy sadist—unsurprising since its source material is Donald Spoto's *Spellbound by Beauty*—this moment of homoerotic tenderness is refreshing, not only because it alleviates the mood of obsessive dread that has dominated the film, but also because it points to the inextricable natures of desire and identification, particularly as Hitchcock experienced them and sought to generate them cinematically in his art. This moment runs counter to the simplistic and relentless public narrative we have been fed that obsessively and *monolithically* returns to Hitchcock's intense desire for blondes, on the one hand, and his wishful identification with his leading men, especially Cary Grant, on the other. This reductive profile is perfectly commensurate with more scholarly accounts of early feminist film theory—primarily Laura Mulvey in her groundbreaking "Visual Pleasure and Narrative Cinema"—where Hitchcock and *Vertigo* are named as practitioner and filmic example of the patriarchal cinematic apparatus that structures classical Hollywood cinema. Mulvey describes an apparatus that privileged the desiring male subject/spectator whose active and authorizing gaze is aligned with both the camera and the (male) protagonist, and directed at the objectified woman, the "bearer-of-the-look." Through this logic, because Woman performs the role of embodying "to-be-looked-at-ness," the female spectator is left unaccounted for, consigned to masochistic identification with the passive woman.[16]

Mulvey has since reformulated some of her descriptions of the workings of the male gaze, most pointedly to make allowances for alternative processes of feminine identification.[17] Yet, insofar as the model of the male gaze and the ideological cinematic apparatus continue to have purchase in film theory, Hitchcock's films, particularly *Vertigo* and *Rear Window*, continue to be regarded as paradigmatic of these gendered processes of reception. This association is unfortunate in its foreclosure on richer, more engaging, and queerer assessments of Hitchcock's apparatus, which, as this chapter argues, allows for great fluidity in gendered identification and desire, just as Hitchcock's own experience of desire and identification was fluid and dynamic. In other words, his aspirational desires and libidinal desires overlapped and informed one another.

Cinematic vicarity: Surrogate versus prosthetic identification

In order to understand better the cognitive and semiotic processes of desire and identification, it is incumbent upon us to achieve a more precise understanding of the language of vicarious experience, upon which the cinema depends for its cognitive, affective, and narrative impressions and effects. Just as in emerging neoliberal discourses, we are to understand *precarity* as the "lived experience of ambient insecurity," I would put forward the usefulness of the term "vicarity" to describe the not-quite-lived experience of surrogate or prosthetic identification.[18] I make a distinction between surrogacy and prosthesis as two different models of vicarious experience in order to stress the variations on vicarity that may represent different relations of identification to desire.

We may describe *surrogate identification* as the imagined inhabiting of the psychic and physical space of another—in the case of cinema, usually the protagonist. For now, I will use the protagonist as the point of cinematic identification, though I concede that identification may happen with different characters, at different times, and with different intensities. In the vicarious experience afforded by the surrogate, the spectator is imaginatively *re-placed* into the diegesis, substituting for, or being substituted by, the subjectivity of the protagonist. Mulvey's initial conception of the male gaze conforms to the surrogate model of identification. Her schema describes the conspiratorial merging of male spectator, camera, and male protagonist to form one penetrating, active male subject who then acts upon or imaginatively possesses the female object. There is a kind of neatness to this model of substitutive identity that I find inimical to the perhaps messier schematizations of identification and desire that structure the Hitchcockian viewing experience.

Prosthetic identification refers to a different relationship between spectator and protagonist (again, for now, simply using the protagonist) that is more complex than simple psychic substitution. It may similarly entail the imaginative inhabiting of the subjectivity of the male protagonist, but it is not a hollowing out of the figure of the other in order to occupy it, so much as a shared, imagined intersubjective experience with the figure of identification. Perhaps one of the most distinctive features of the prosthetic identification that I propose is that the figure of identification is aestheticized, rendered as an object of sorts, while retaining an imagined, shared agency and consciousness. As the term suggests, the spectator's relation is not substitutive, but prosthetic, a psychic and physical extension of the spectator, who is in turn transformed and redeemed by him, providing identificatory pleasure. The prosthetic connection to the protagonist is an eroticized one, in that frisson produced by the dual corporeal inhabitation and shared subjectivity, pleasurably tests its boundaries.

It is my contention that, whereas Hitchcock's cinema is often described as fostering a sense of surrogate identification, his dynamic sense of play with the camera, his elaborate configurations of point of view, and his orchestration of often unpredictable sympathies and antipathies toward both male and female characters encourage a variety of prosthetic identifications. In labeling this process "prosthetic," the concept of the dildonic may arise as sexual (and likely phallic) extension of the spectator, but I would argue that prosthesis could refer to any number of body parts—eyes, hands, shoulders—and bodily accouterments—armor, weapon, mask—that produce an enhanced or heightened sense of diegetic self on the part of the spectator.

One Hitchcockian film example that illustrates a facilitation of prosthetic identification occurs in *Notorious* (1946), in a famous love scene between Alicia (Ingrid Bergman) and Devlin (Cary Grant). Devlin and Alicia have just returned home to their apartment, where Alicia proposes to make them a chicken dinner. As they begin to embrace, the camera captures them in a medium two-shot, and it slowly pushes in to frame them in a medium close-up two-shot. In order to circumvent the Production Code which disallowed prolonged scenes of kissing, Hitchcock had them intersperse their kisses with small talk about their meal (prompting writer Ben Hecht, upon seeing the scene, to bark, "I don't get all this talk about chicken!").[19] As the couple walks across the floor toward the telephone, the camera tracks them, maintaining the medium close-up from start to finish, while managing to change their left-right orientation through angle in the continuous shot. When asked by Truffaut to comment on his choices in this scene, Hitchcock responded:

> I conceived that scene in terms of the participants' desire not to interrupt the romantic moment. . . . Had they broken apart, all of the emotion would have been dissipated. . . . I also felt that the public, represented by the camera, was the third party to this embrace. The public was being given the great privilege of embracing Cary Grant and Ingrid Bergman together. It was a kind of temporary ménage a trois.[20]

Far from the conventionally gendered alignment of subject and object, Hitchcock's camera and its vantage point constitute a third element, which can be imaginatively taken up by the desiring spectator. Several different configurations of erotic syntax may emerge from this filmic arrangement. Let us assume that Hitchcock, in this scenario is not only director, but spectator. We may parse the syntax variously:

1. (Subject) Hitchcock + (Subject) Devlin—(desire/possess)→(Object) Alicia
2. (Subject) Hitchcock + (Subject) Alicia—(desire/possess)→(Object) Devlin
3. (Subject) Hitchcock—(desires/possesses)→(Object) Devlin + (Object) Alicia
4. (Subject) Hitchcock—(desires/possesses)→(Direct Object) Alicia~~(Indirect Object) Devlin

5 (Subject) Hitchcock—(desires/possesses)→(Direct Object) Devlin~~(Indirect Object) Alicia.

6 (Sub/Ob) Hitchcock—(desires/possesses)→(Sub/Ob) Devlin—(desires/ possesses)→(Sub/Ob) Alicia—(desires/possesses)→(Sub/Ob) Hitchcock...

7 (Subject) Hitchcock—identifies with→(Predicate Nominative) Love/ Desire—Between→(Object) Alicia and (Object) Devlin (an ambient identification)

The multitude of viewing positions, of identificatory points of entry, and of possible objects and subjects of desire belies any simple model of the male gaze. The queer playfulness of the configurations made possible through his dispersal of potential vantage points across gender and syntactic position demonstrate the refusal of monolithic libidinal investment.

Chapter 3 explored the possibilities of Hitchcock's own identifications with his female characters, particularly through his sympathies with their desires for love and the acts of consumption that demonstrate or emblematize that love. John Russell Taylor, in his biography *Hitch*, similarly suggests that, because of his female leads' cool aloofness, contrasted with their yearning to express passion, "It was actually his heroines that he identified with." This cross-gender identification on the part of the director further indicts the inflexibility of the male subject-female object dichotomy in the model of the patriarchal cinematic apparatus.

Hitchcock's relation to filmic (and cultural) masculinity also suggests a queer (if not gay) aesthetic. His admiration for and envy of strong masculine beauty contained inflections of desire, as dramatized in *The Girl*'s homoerotic encounter between Hitchcock and Brown. His aesthetic relation to male beauty rested on a semiotic of naturalness, ruggedness, transparency, and authenticity. While he attributed performativity and masquerade to female beauty—thus, his obsessive attention to costume, jewelry, hair, makeup, and other feminine accessories—his stance on the male beauties he directed was typically, "Do nothing." Once, when Gregory Peck asked how he should be playing a certain scene, Hitchcock responded, "Blankly." Peck took this as disinterest in his performance, and Spoto has suggested that his purported lack of direction for male actors was rooted in his envy of them.

I suggest, however, that responses like these revealed a belief on Hitchcock's part, first of all, that affect could be manufactured through montage in the editing room; but more importantly, they revealed a belief that masculine beauty was best left unadorned, understated, precisely because of its power, and his reticence to coach or manipulate male performance actually signaled his reluctance to render it "obvious" and therefore cheapen it. He famously stated, "Cary Grant was the only actor I ever loved," and he would often praise Grant for his naturalness and self-sufficiency in assessments like "Cary is marvelous, you see. One doesn't direct Cary Grant; one simply puts him in front of the camera."[21] Eva Marie Saint recalls in an interview, that Hitchcock only had three pieces of acting advice to offer her: "1. Lower your voice. 2. Don't use your hands, and 3. Always look Cary in the eyes."[22] This advice importantly reveals Hitchcock's investment in the female gaze, and the male as potential object of desire, at least in this context. Hitchcock expressed similar feelings for Leo G. Carroll, whom he employed many times, calling him "the perfect screen actor" who brought "nothing to his part except himself."[23]

James Stewart expressed anxiety about the sort of transparency and naturalness that Hitchcock expected of him. After Hitch told him to "Be yourself" in response to a question about character motivation, Stewart mused, "That's the toughest thing anyone could ever ask me to do. No cover. Go out there naked as James Stewart. I mean, what do you do with your hands?" It seems not to have occurred to the director that these men he idealized may also have vulnerabilities and insecurities about their performance, and that they were *performing* masculinity, not *exuding* it. Hitchcock clearly dis-identified with this rugged, natural masculinity. He identified with the performative expectations of women, and never appeared in public without an immaculate suit, a dramatic or humorous conceit, an anecdote, gimmick, or prop for support. The masculine self-sufficiency he coveted was never available to him, though his desire for and fantasmatic identification with his leading men soothed these feelings of inadequacy about his own unacceptable body, if only momentarily and vicariously.

The Tickles: Subjectivities without bodies

In a 1964 interview on *Telescope*, host Fletcher Markle asked Hitchcock to predict the status of cultural entertainment in the year 3000. Hitchcock proceeded with an elaborate description, first issuing the fascinating proviso, "If there is still a need for entertainment." His imaginative account proceeds thusly:

> In the distant future they will have what I call "the Tickles." People will go into a big darkened auditorium and they will be mass-hypnotized. Instead of identifying themselves with the characters on screen, they will be that character, and when they buy their ticket, they will be able to choose which

> character to be. They will suffer all of the agonies and enjoy the romance with a beautiful woman or handsome man. I call them "the Tickles" because when a character is tickled, the audience will feel it. Then, the lights come up and it's all over.[24]

What is of particular interest in Hitchcock's account of the future is the anticipation that as a culture we will have moved "beyond" identification. At first glance, his depiction sounds like simple surrogate identification, whereby we are "replaced" by the character—her perspective and subjectivity—for the duration of the performance/hypnosis.

Yet, something queerer is at stake in Hitchcock's forecasting the disappearance of identification. If cinematic identification is the cognitive equivalent of the sentence, "I am like you," or "I think that I am you (provisionally)," the Tickles, as Hitchcock has framed it, effaces the "I" subject, whereby it dissolves to or ontologically yields to the subjectivity of the character. One important difference between surrogate identification and the Tickles is that when we identify a character as our surrogate, we focus on that character, yet our viewing is filtered through our concomitant awareness of, and analogizing of, our extra-filmic self, however much we downplay the intrusive voice of "reality" that makes full absorption impossible. As Hitchcock conceives the Tickles, however, the spectator's self and her body seem to cede their status as the ultimate referent, and the occupation of a character is neither intersubjective nor recognizably self-conscious.

What Hitchcock really reveals here in this interview is the fantasy of the eradication of the spectatorial body. The premise of grounding desire and identification in the denial of the body of the original subject throws a queer wrench into the heteronormative assumptions about how desires proceed rationally from embodied identities. As a fat man in a world that placed an extravagant premium on fitness and masculine beauty, the director must have experienced this queer erasure of the subject's body as a seductive notion. In an ecosystem that trafficked in subjectivities without bodies as original referents, he could enjoy pleasures untainted by the shame of the excesses that marked his body and could not ultimately be exorcized through surrogacy or prosthesis. This disembodied subjectivity, of course, is the stuff of fantasy, but it registers a poetic desire for a liberating corporeal annihilation, where cultural signification could be stripped away to reveal a self that was neither fat nor thin—a self that became what it desired, and loved what it became.

Epilogue

Hitchcock and his works continue to experience life among generation Y and beyond, though it is admittedly disconcerting to walk into an undergraduate lecture hall and see few, if any, lights go on at the mention of his name. Disconcerting as it may be, all ill feelings are forgotten when I watch an auditorium of eighteen- to twenty-one-year-olds transported by the emotions, the humor, and the compulsions of his cinema. But certainly the college classroom is not the only guardian of Hitchcock's flame. His films still play at retrospectives, in film festivals, in the rising number of film studies classes in high schools, on Turner Classic Movies, and other networks devoted to the "oldies." The wonderful *Bates Motel* has emerged as a TV serial prequel to *Psycho*, illustrating the formative years of Norman Bates; it will see a second season in the coming months. *Alfred Hitchcock Presents* and *The Alfred Hitchcock Hour* are still in strong syndication. Both his films and television shows do very well in collections and singly on Amazon and other e-commerce sites. And as I have learned many times over, grandparents and parents growing up in the 1940s through the 1960s love telling their children about their first time watching *Psycho*'s shower scene and about their deep distrust of birds after cringing through his follow-up.

The year 2012 saw the release of two Hitchcock biopics that were reasonably successful, both critically and commercially—one in wide cinematic release and the other as a made-for-TV movie on HBO. The two films, *Hitchcock* and *The Girl*, focus on the making of *Psycho* and the Hitchcock-Hedren relationship during *The Birds* and *Marnie*, respectively. I use "biopic" advisedly because each covers a very small section of Hitchcock's life and work (more a "slice of life" than a "piece of cake," perhaps, and slices that should not necessarily be extrapolated), and *The Girl* especially is arguable in its status as a biopic in that it privileges Hedren's point of view over her director's. I would like to end this book with a brief consideration of these two films and how they will potentially help shape the public memory of Hitchcock, especially in light of his appetites, which are both the overarching concern of this book and the focus of the biopics, albeit in quite different ways.

Hitchcock was produced by Fox Searchlight and released in November 2012. Directed by Sacha Gervasi, a first-time feature director, the film stars Anthony Hopkins as Alfred Hitchcock, Helen Mirren as wife Alma, and Scarlett Johanssen as Janet Leigh, with a wonderful supporting cast including, among others, Jessica Biel as Vera Miles, Toni Collette as longtime collaborator and assistant Peggy Robertson, and an impeccable James D'Arcy as Anthony Perkins. The screenplay was written by John J. McLaughlin, who used Stephen Rebello's book *Alfred Hitchcock and the Making of Psycho* as source material.

The film opens with Hitchcock's reluctant consideration of Robert Bloch's bestselling novel *Psycho* for his next movie. He has just come off the wildly successful *North by Northwest*, which he made for MGM, and he faces still one more film as a contractual obligation to Paramount. The film takes us through Hitch's growing fascination with the story, and his various struggles with Paramount and the censoring arm of Geoffrey Shurlock's enforcement of the Production Code to get *Psycho* made, his marital struggles—in terms of their budgetary crises and Alma's extramarital interests—and his usual battles with food, drink, and blonde leading ladies. The film ending is straight out of Hollywood: Alma recommits to the Hitchcock marriage and collaboration, Hitch creates a wildly successful film, and Janet Leigh escapes with only minor trauma. The most interesting thing about the film from a narrative perspective is its beginning with a reenactment of serial killer Ed Geins's murder of his brother (who has just called him a Mama's Boy), and the interspersed passages throughout the film that dramatize Hitchcock's fantasized interactions with Ed Gein. While these fantasies seem to read as moments when the director is trying to get inside the head of his next lead character, there's a comic reversal that takes place, which puts Hitchcock on the analyst couch and Gein in the place of therapist, and we come to realize that Hitch's creation has in turn begun to probe the director's own dark thoughts about his mother, about sexuality, and about aggression.

The Girl—a Warner Brothers-BBC-HBO collaboration—picks up almost exactly where *Hitchcock* leaves off, chronologically speaking. Written by Gwyneth Hughes, who used Donald Spoto's *Spellbound by Beauty* as its source material, and directed by Julian Jerrold, *The Girl* features Sienna Miller as Tippi Hedren, Toby Jones as Hitchcock, Imelda Staunton as Alma, and an impressive supporting cast of Conrad Kemp's Evan Hunter, Penelope Wilton's Peggy Robertson, and Carl Beukes's Jim Brown. The movie debuted on HBO on October 20, just two weeks before the theatrical release of *Hitchcock*. The film takes us from the discovery (by Alma) of Tippi Hedren, her subsequent casting, all the way through the productions of both *The Birds* and *Marnie*. As mentioned above, the film champions Hedren's point of view, while Hitchcock is presented as the film's principal antagonist—a man desperate for the love and attentions of Hedren and sadistically cruel to her when these feelings are not returned. It is a film about the abuse of power and the psychological trauma such abuse inflicts, particularly when the abuser is a rich white man who is universally loved and respected, and never questioned.

The interpretation of Alfred Hitchcock's character is markedly different in each film. Hopkins's Hitchcock is something of an overgrown child, an indulgent imp, given to late night caviar binges and secreting liquor in magazine stands, and Mirren portrays Alma as an aggressive, savvy writer, networker, and perhaps most intriguingly, as a nanny of sorts to her husband—the one with the power to bestow foie gras and take it away. Their sparring is fun, superficially wounding, and indicative of a comfortable familiarity, and a mutual ability to provoke and inspire. Hopkins studied hard and well for the part, replicating Hitchcock's awkward mannerisms, his tendency to gulp down drink, whether wine or brandy, and his delight in feeding delicious crumbs to the media. Toby Jones's Hitchcock is more reserved and sullen, more malicious and nasty in his pursuit of an intended effect, whether from wife, would-be lover, or underling. Imelda Staunton's Alma is more passive than Mirren's, more resigned to Hitchcock's flaws than combative about them, and ultimately a much sadder woman. If Hopkins and Mirren engage in sparring of wits, Jones and Staunton are often out for blood, *Who's Afraid of Virginia Woolf*-style. In *Hitchcock,* we see a man bewitched by food and by women. In fact, he is eating in the majority of scenes in which he is featured. *The Girl*'s Hitch is almost never seen eating, but almost always drinking heavily; two scenes portray a stuporously drunk Hitchcock, who is filled with frustrated desire (mostly for Hedren and perhaps a little for Jim Brown) and self-loathing. All in all, *The Girl* has the stamp of Spoto's recriminations on it; it portrays Hitchcock as defeated by his compulsions and dangerous to those under his care. *Hitchcock,* on the other hand, has been justifiably accused of tidying up the messier bits of biography but, to its credit, it depicts how his appetites and his artistic drive fed one another.

I applaud *The Girl* for making visible a story of exploitation and abuse that had been papered over by so many layers of denial, by power-saturated conspiracies of silence, and fear of reprisals in an environment historically hostile to women. Implicitly argued in this movie is that artistic genius and immense power do not exempt one from moral culpabilities, that one's greatness does not license lechery or deep injury. Yet, by and large, *The Girl* suggests that Hitchcock's sadism toward women was something he was both conscious and unrepentant of—that his actions toward females came from a fundamental place of wishing them harm and humiliation. Born a decade or so after *The Birds*, I can only speculate. Yet, I find it very hard to believe that, in regard to filming the upstairs bird attack with Hedren, throughout what would have to have been one of the most exhilarating days of shooting, Hitchcock remained immobile in his director's chair, leering and seething with hatred at Hedren, rather than engaging with the shifting camera setups, the difficulties in preserving continuity, and the other similar wonderful technical challenges presented by the scene. The most humane moment we get from the director in the film is a muted, momentary expression of regret on his face after Hedren has been reduced to a prostrate mess.

As this book makes clear, a contemplation of Hitchcock's appetites makes a picture of the man and the artist more complete, more intimate, and more human. Taken together, these films reveal a talented artist and a man of many appetites. Depending on which representation compels us more, we come away contemplating a man either destroyed by, or destructive in, his unsatisfied hungers or a man-boy who progressed through life in cycles of indulgence, inappropriateness, and profound creativity. Truthfully, neither film leaves me with the Hitchcock I have known through his films, though I strongly believe and hope that future audiences will come to know him better through his own work, than through these biographical representations.

I will close with a quick story that exemplifies how I like to remember Hitchcock. It is about *Rope*, and I call it *The Parable of the Paté*. Housekeeper Mrs. Wilson (Edith Evanson) enters Philip and Brandon's apartment after a day of shopping for their party that evening. Flushed, she claims to have traveled to five delis just to get the right paté. She ends up securing the product at a deli frequented by Jimmy Stewart's Rupert Cadell—a man for whom she has giddy feelings. If Mirren's Alma in *Hitchcock* functions as the keeper of the paté, Mrs. Wilson takes on the mantle in *Rope* in a fine and energetic fashion. At one moment, she uses the store-bought paté to attempt to cozy up to Rupert, and she is rebuffed with a joke. Twice, she warns Philip (Farley Granger), "You're too skinny," and "Don't let them gobble up all that paté before you get to it." The guilty as sin Philip, who has just murdered a friend and served dinner from where his body is stashed, taking the lead from his lover Brandon (John Dall), never gets to the paté, though he manages to consume a number of martinis and highballs throughout the party. Finally, in her last act of paté-enforcement, Mrs. Wilson creeps up behind Janet Walker (Joan Chandler), a smart and stubborn society girl who writes a column about keeping the body beautiful, and cautions, "If I were you, I'd go easy on the paté, dear. Calories . . ."

When I watch these scenes, I laugh, and I imagine Hitchcock's dividing his identifications between Philip and Janet. Hitchcock surely felt an affinity with Philip, the golden child, the up-and-coming virtuoso with special talents, who has learned entitlement through being coddled and pampered, though never fully comfortable with the attentions, as they may unearth more than he is willing to share. And then there is Janet, the affable gal who plays the part she is supposed to, is appropriately ironic about her patriarchally aligned advice column, and who has an appetite that gets checked and is left unsatisfied. Between a character whose appetite is spoiled by the knowledge of his self-loathing deeds and one whose appetite remains unsatisfied to conform to the "body beautiful" that is her bread-and-butter, the paté goes tragically uneaten.

First, I like to think of this motif as Hitchcock's acknowledgment of unfortunate disparities in the social treatment of men and women—remember, this is Hitchcock as I *like* to remember him, so projection may be included. Mrs. Wilson is then not just a guardian of paté, but also a custodian of appropriate gender roles. Under her watchful gaze, the cultural permissiveness toward men spoils them, and the expectations on women are painfully unreasonable. When I watch the exchange between Mrs. Wilson and Janet, I always immediately remember a line by comedienne Janeane Garofalo: "Women are often their own greatest enemy, but I still blame men." Secondly, I see Hitchcock in these two characters because he was surrounded by permissiveness—he was wealthy, respected, rewarded for his creativity—yet could not indulge in certain pleasures (sexual ones, especially) and often could not enjoy his indulgences (gulping his food and drink), whether because of his loyalty to Alma, his embarrassment around the physical experience of pleasure, or his great contempt for his own body.

Paté or no paté, life is not without its consolatory pleasures, both for Hitchcock and for his Janet and Philip (though we may question the pleasures in Philip's future). Thankfully for us, Hitchcock was always more conversant in the idiom of cinematic pleasures than he was in the ones that surfaced in his own life. And it is these pleasures, the creation and satisfaction of these appetites—decadent, stimulating, renewing, and joyful—that comprise his cinematic legacy.

Notes

Introduction

1 Alfred Hitchcock, from "After-Dinner Speech" at the Screen Producers Guild Dinner, Los Angeles, March 7, 1965.

2 John Russell Taylor, *Hitch: The Life and Times of Alfred Hitchcock* (New York: Da Capo Press, 1996), 17.

3 Jan Olsson's recent book *Hitchcock a la Carte* (Durham: Duke University Press, 2015) similarly investigates Hitchcock's size as both an integral part of his self-promotion as a celebrity and as a compelling factor in the analysis of his use of food in his two television series *Alfred Hitchcock Presents* and *The Alfred Hitchcock Hour.*

4 Charlotte Chandler, *It's Only a Movie: Alfred Hitchcock, a Personal Biography* (New York: Simon & Schuster, 2005), 11.

5 Ibid., 11.

6 Sander Gilman, *Fat Boys* (Lincoln: University of Nebraska Press, 2004), 11.

7 Chapter 5 contains a more in-depth look at Hitchcock's childhood relationships.

8 Chandler, *It's Only*, 33.

9 Donald Spoto, *The Dark Side of Genius: The Life of Alfred Hitchcock* (New York: Da Capo Press, 1999), 171.

10 Details of his diet and weight gain, and also the public reportage of his diet, can be found in greater detail in Chapter 1.

11 Pat Hitchcock O' Connell and Laurent Bouzereau, *Alma Hitchcock: The Woman Behind the Man* (New York: Berkley Book, 2003), 184.

12 Ibid., 256–84.

13 Ibid., 229.

14 William Rothman, *Hitchcock: The Murderous Gaze* (Cambridge, MA: Harvard University Press, 1982), 106.

15 Tania Modleski, *The Women Who Knew Too Much: Hitchcock and Feminist Theory* (New York: Routledge, 2005).

16 Laura Mulvey, "Visual Pleasure and Narrative Cinema," *Screen* 16, no. 3 (Spring, 1975): 6–18.

17 Modleski, *Women*, 7.

Chapter 1

1 By "spectacular" here, I emphasize the notion of body-as-spectacle, not a degree of fatness.

2 Patrick McGilligan, *Alfred Hitchcock: A Life in Darkness and Light* (New York: Regan/Harper Collins, 2003).

3 Donald Spoto, *The Dark Side of Genius: The Life of Alfred Hitchcock* (New York: Da Capo Press, 1999), 170–71.

4 McGilligan, *Darkness and Light*, 205.

5 All telegrams, memos, and letters in this chapter are archived in the David O. Selznick collection in the Harry Ransom Center in Austin, Texas, from which I received a generous fellowship for the summer of 2012 to research this first chapter of the book. I cannot thank the Ransom Center staff enough for their help and support.

6 Memo, Selznick Archive.

7 Katharine Roberts, "Mystery Man: Thrills and Chills of Alfred Hitchcock," *Collier's Weekly* (August 5, 1939): 22.

8 Obviously, we can never be certain that Hitchcock's diet regimens were as strict or consistently followed as his public reportage of them suggests. McGilligan and Spoto both comment on episodes of "cheating" on his diet(s) in the early 1940s. Regardless of the accuracy of his dietary claims, he nevertheless wanted to convey a sense of commitment to improving his body.

9 Alfred Hitchcock, "The Woman Who Knows Too Much," *McCall's* 83 (March, 1956): 12, 14.

10 Spoto, *Dark Side*, 234–35.

11 Michael Balcon, *London Sunday Dispatch*, August 25, 1940.

12 Hitchcock struck back at Balcon in the press.

> Balcon's view is colored by his own personal experiences with Hollywood, which have invariably wound up unfortunately for Balcon. . . . We have all placed ourselves at the disposal of our government. . . . The British government has only to call on me for my services. The manner in which I am helping my country is not Mr. Balcon's business. Hitchcock, Alfred. ("Hitchcock Responds to 'Deserter' Charge," *New York World-Telegram*, August 27, 1940)

13 McGilligan, *Darkness and Light*.

14 Hitchcock's venture with Bernstein Transatlantic Pictures was short-lived. They only made two pictures together, *Rope* (1948) and *Under Capricorn* (1949); neither performed well at the box office. The company sank into oblivion the following year during the filming of *Stage Fright*, and Warner Brothers/First National had to come to the aid of the production to finance and release it. This was the end of Transatlantic, and the beginning of Hitchcock's lucrative deals with Warner for the first half of the 1950s.

15 Alva Johnston, "300-Pound Prophet Comes to Hollywood," *Saturday Evening Post* 215, no. 47 (May 22, 1943): 12.

16 Myron Selznick Archive, File 169, Folder 3, Harry Ransom Center, Austin, Texas.

17 Ibid.

18 Ibid.

19 He was also offered a job as producer and MC of the Pabst Blue Ribbon Beer show, another DeMille-like role, and also for the Philip Morris Playhouse.

20 Here, and in the paragraphs that follow, the italicized words and phrases are my emphasis. I use them to foreground the language of fatness that occurs with great frequency in SIP communications.

21 An assumption that underwrites this entire book is that American culture, and to some degree Western culture in general, is fat-phobic. Fat bodies are devalued for their failure to uphold normative standards of size. Furthermore, American culture conditions its subjects to link attractiveness and desirability, even acceptability, to the maintenance of fit bodies. Thus, Selznick and colleagues' fat-phobia is not an allegation that sets them apart from most of the populace; it simply manifests itself in an important and germane way in the relationship with Hitchcock.

22 After *Foreign Correspondent*, Selznick worried that Wanger was complaining around town that Hitchcock was slow in shooting, and feared that it would hurt his reputation. Also, in 1946, he angrily decried Hitch's "increasing habit of taking a year per picture."

23 Rene Clair's first American film *The Flame of New Orleans* (1941) for Universal performed disastrously at the box office, so much so that his career was in jeopardy. Through *I Married a Witch* (1942) and *It Happened Tomorrow* (1944), and especially with the success of *And Then There Were None* (1945), he fought his way back to respectability. While Jean Renoir's first American films, *Swamp Water* (1941) and *This Land Is Mine* (1943), made a profit, he struggled a great deal finding an acceptable project in Hollywood and also had great difficulty adapting to American filming techniques.

24 Spoto mentions in *Dark Side of Genius* that in his 1939 Christmas holiday card to Hitchcock, Selznick gently offered some nutrition pointers, in acknowledgment of concerns with his weight. That one correspondence is the only time I have heard of or seen any encouragement by Selznick for him to lose weight.

25 Right after this slight, Selznick had his opportunity to return the favor. Hoping to draw on elements from *Spellbound* to form the backbone of one of his *Hitchcock Presents*, Hitchcock petitioned him for use of the story, and then-owner of the film Selznick refused him.

Chapter 2

1 According to Janet Staiger in her essay, "Creating the Brand: Hitchcock's Touch," (in *The Cambridge American Companion to Hitchcock*, ed. Jonathan Freeman), the *Young and Innocent* cameo, was reproduced in Leslie Perkoff's "The Censor and Sydney Street," *World Film News* 2, no. 12

(March 1938): 4–5. The same image appeared in the Hellman profile on him in *Life*, November 20, 1939, where the cutline introduced the idea that Hitchcock liked to be in one scene in each of his movies. Staiger reads that image not as Hitchcock as a mere spectator but as a journalist attempting to snap a photo of our "wrong man" being led out of the courthouse.

2 David Sterritt, *The Films of Alfred Hitchcock* (Boston: Cambridge University Press, 1993), 11–16.

3 Tom Ryall, *Alfred Hitchcock & the British Cinema* (Urbana: University of Illinois Press, 1986), 165. Ronald Christ, "*Strangers on a Train*: The Pattern of Encounter," in *Focus on Hitchcock*, ed. Albert LaValley (New York: Prentice Hall, 1972), 107.

4 Sterritt, *Alfred Hitchcock*, 12.

5 I concede that spectators watch film with differing degrees of concentration, and are differently susceptible to diegetic disruption; while some may greet Hitchcock's presence with a minimal feeling of dissonance, others may feel disengaged from the story in a more profound way. I still call the cameo an avoidance of total diegetic disruption because the average viewer becomes reabsorbed quickly into the narrative.

6 I would like to thank Janet Staiger for helping me think through the mesogetic as a narrative mode versus intertextuality as a reading strategy.

7 Obviously, this was not Hitchcock's first picture but, as indicated in the first chapter, it was the first great success of his career, and the idea of an "origin story" for the cameos is heightened with this description.

8 This passage about Hitchcock's cameos was written by Hitch to Jack Goldstein of Vanguard Films, in a letter dated October 19, 1945. Vanguard coproduced *Spellbound* with SIP.

9 This was the original plan for his cameo. He ended up showing us the back of his head in an editorial room of the newspaper, and then later as part of the mob surrounding the Lodger.

10 I use "material" here with a dual meaning—the cliché, but also the reference to the materialism of the body in contrast with his interior sense of self.

11 Sterritt, *Alfred Hitchcock*, 12.

12 Technically, Hitchcock's appearance in *The Wrong Man* is longer, but people do not consider that a typical cameo, and for good reason, as Hitch addresses the audience directly, before the "film" starts, closer to the format of his *Alfred Hitchcock Presents* appearances.

13 Sterritt incorrectly identifies the scene as taking place on a bus.

14 Charlotte Chandler, *It's Only a Movie: Alfred Hitchcock, a Personal Biography* (New York: Simon & Schuster, 2005), 33–34.

15 Sterritt, *Alfred Hitchcock*, 13.

16 Tania Modleski, *The Women Who Knew Too Much: Hitchcock and Feminist* Theory (New York: Routledge, 2005), 27.

17 Ibid.

18 Ibid.

19 In *Shadow of a Doubt*, we also have a couple bound together by secret knowledge. Yet, rather than the sense of coercion that characterizes Frank and Alice's relationship in *Blackmail*, Jack's willingness to keep Charlie's secret—again, a triumph of love over duty—manifests his abiding love for and understanding of her.

20 Sterritt describes Cotten's Charlie rising "like a vampire from his coffin." (Sterritt, *Alfred Hitchcock*, 54).

21 John Steinbeck, Jo Swerling, and Ben Hecht (uncredited) wrote the screenplay for *Lifeboat*.

22 Anthony Schaffer wrote the screenplay of *Frenzy*, adapting it from the novel *Goodbye Piccadilly, Farewell Leicester Square* by Arthur La Bern.

23 Chandler, *It's Only*, 152.

24 By "main character," I mean one who is of consequence to the story, either a lead or supporting actor, not an extra.

25 In these contexts of the cameo, I use "interaction" to refer to eye contact, and acknowledgment, not necessarily mutual.

26 Hitchcock's use of "MacGuffin" here is somewhat puzzling. Obviously, elsewhere, he uses "MacGuffin" to describe a plot point that is of great interest to the main characters, but ultimately is of little consequence for the viewer. In this instance, it seems that Hitchcock is jokingly referring to "MacGuffin" as a kind of animal, in opposition to "ham," the meat of a pig. Continuing the sandwich metaphor, he indicates that the "meat" of his sandwich is simply a performance that is ultimately of little consequence to the story. Though the appearance is, according to Hitchcock's analogy, but a trifle, it participates in the trope of theatricality, as it captures a "failed performance."

27 The world of performance is depicted in several other Hitchcock films: modeling in *The Lodger* (1927); the circus in *Murder!* (1930); and again, though briefly, in *Saboteur* (1942); a movie theater in *Sabotage* (1936); the world of musical celebrity in *The Man Who Knew Too Much* (1956); and tennis celebrity in *Strangers on a Train* (1951).

28 I say "that made it into the released film" because several cameo scenes were written, some committed to film, before they were scrapped. One such example was a cameo scene in *Saboteur* (1942), where Hitch and Dorothy Parker were shot crossing a city street in mid-quarrel, though it was possibly deemed too intrusive into the narrative. Instead, we get just a brief glimpse of him standing in front of a drug store an hour into the film.

29 Many spectators have incorrectly assumed that Hitch breaks the fourth wall in this scene, looking directly into the camera, but in actuality, he is simply making eye contact with the character.

30 I am going to assume that audiences were supposed to gather that actual musical instruments were to be found inside. In an intro to one episode of *Alfred Hitchcock Presents*, Hitchcock carries a violin case that in fact has a machine gun inside. As he fires it, musical notes come out.

31 The quotation is cited in many different publications, though its first expression is not documented.

32 See, for instance, the excellent article "Criss-Cross: Paranoia and Projection in *Strangers on a Train*," in Alexander Doty and Corey Creekmur's *Out in Culture: Gay, Lesbian and Queer Essays on Popular Culture*, ed. Sabrina Barton (London and Durham: Duke University Press, 1995), 216–38.

33 Conversation with Norman Holland, e-mail, January 8, 2009.

34 By "comic," I refer to a comedic moment present in the diegesis itself, not simply in the comedy the audience may derive from the cameo's diegetic confusion.

Chapter 3

1 "A Talk with Hitchcock," *Telescope*, hosted and produced by Fletcher Markle, January 1, 1964.

2 Donald Spoto, *The Dark Side of Genius: The Life of Alfred Hitchcock* (New York: Da Capo Press, 1983), 82.

3 Patrick McGilligan, *Alfred Hitchcock: A Life in Darkness and Light* (New York: Regan/Harper Collins, 2003), 26.

4 Ibid., 177.

5 http://productioncode.dhwritings.com/multipleframes_productioncode.php.

6 The Code was in effect before 1933, but was not systematically enforced until Joe Breen took command of the office, requiring script approval for all Hollywood releases.

7 I am indebted to the Harry Ransom Center's Selznick collection, where I was able to read the various incarnations of the *Notorious* script.

8 The finished film does not depict the death of Alicia, though her fate is uncertain, as the final shot captures Devlin and the barely conscious Alicia's escape by car.

9 Donald Spoto, *The Art of Alfred Hitchcock: Fifty Years of his Motion Pictures* (New York: Anchor Books, 1976), 155.

10 Originally published in *Film Weekly* (September 20, 1935): 10.

11 Barbara J. Buchanan, "Women Are a Nuisance," in *Film Weekly* (September 20, 1935): 10. Reprinted in *Hitchcock on Hitchcock*, ed. Sidney Gottlieb (Berkeley: University of California Press, 1995), 80–81.

12 Spoto, *Dark Side*, 82.

13 H. E. F. Donohue, "Remembrance of Murders Past: An Interview with Alfred Hitchcock," *The New York Times*.

14 Also titled *Dangerous Virtue*, *The Prude's Fall* (1924) credited Hitchcock as Writer, Art Director, and Assistant Director.

15 Donohue, "Remembrance."

16 Cognac is a distilled form of brandy; the two are often conflated by Hitchcock, and by American culture at large.

17 Observed by his lead Joel McCrea, and recorded in McGilligan's *A Life in Darkness and Light*.

18 Spoto, *Dark Side*, 382.

19 Ibid.

20 Charlotte Chandler, *It's Only a Movie: Alfred Hitchcock, a Personal Biography* (New York: Simon & Schuster, 2005), 1.

21 The same joke is used a year later in director W. S. Van Dyke's *Shadow of the Thin Man*, when loveable alcoholic Nick Charles is dared by his wife to forgo his usual martini in favor of a full glass of milk, which he distastefully downs, as mystified wife, son, and maid look on. He too observes that the milk tastes "like poison."

22 Michael Walker, *Hitchcock's Motifs* (Amsterdam: Amsterdam University Press, 2005), 30.

23 Walker also comments that in *Psycho*, the milk Norman serves Marion is "tainted" after Mrs. Bates is heard castigating Norman for attempting to satisfy Marion's "ugly appetites."

24 Mikhail Bakhtin, *Rabelais and His World* (Bloomington: Indiana University Press, 1965), 10.

25 All the audience knows in that regard is that the child likely does not belong to Guy.

26 Nine characters are victims of strangulation in Hitchcock's films—six women and three men. The method of killing was appealing to Hitchcock, perhaps, because it is so intimate, consummately cinematic (in terms of opportunities for POV), and provides the drama of life slowly leaving the body. It is interesting to consider the throat as conduit for both air and food/drink. Strangulation is the violent occlusion of both processes.

27 Francois Truffaut first made this observation of Hitch's filmmaking during their famous interview of 1964. Hitchcock liked this formulation and used it often afterward.

28 David Sterritt, *The Films of Alfred Hitchcock* (New York: Cambridge University Press, 1993), 16.

29 In the original script, Eve says, "I never make love on an empty stomach," but the line failed to meet with the censor's approval, so they changed the verb to "discuss."

30 Francois Truffaut, *Hitchcock/Truffaut*, ed. Francois Truffaut (New York: Simon & Schuster, 1983), 201.

31 Tania Modleski, *The Women Who Knew Too Much: Hitchcock and Feminist Theory* (New York: Routledge, 2005), 108.

32 Ibid.

33 Walker, *Motifs*, 183. Walker's book contains a fascinating discussion of the Hitchcock meal scene as a site for the examination of male sexual inadequacy and female dis-ease.

34 Truffaut, *Hitchcock*, 320.

35 Ibid.

Chapter 4

1 Laura Mulvey, "Visual Pleasure and Narrative Cinema," *Screen* 16, no. 3 (Spring 1975): 6–18.

2 Francois Truffaut, ed., *Hitchcock/Truffaut: The Definitive Study of Alfred Hitchcock* (New York: Simon & Schuster, 1983), 222.

3 Patrick McGilligan, *Alfred Hitchcock: A Life in Darkness and Light* (New York: Regan/Harper Collins, 2003), 486.

4 John Russell Taylor, *Hitch: The Life and Times of Alfred Hitchcock* (Boston: DaCapo Press), 1978.

5 Jean Douchet, "Hitch et son public," *Cahiers du Cinema* 19, no. 3 (1960): 10.

6 Robert Stam and Roberta Pearson, "Hitchcock's *Rear Window*: Reflexivity and the Critique of Voyeurism," *Enclitic* 7, no. 1 (Spring, 1983): 143.

7 I am assuming that Miss Torso and Stanley are not married because she does not wear a wedding ring—the film's plot hinges so strongly on the notion that all women wear their wedding rings, it would seem strange for her not to. Thus, when Stanley says, "Boy, it's good to be home," I take home to mean New York City after his army service ended, not the apartment in particular.

8 Stam and Pearson, "Reflexivity," 201.

9 Zora Neale Hurston, *Their Eyes Were Watching God* (New York: Harper Perennial, 1990), 3.

10 Truffaut, *Hitchcock*, 216.

11 Robin Wood, *Hitchcock's Films Revisited* (New York: Columbia University Press, 1989), 103.

12 Truffaut, *Hitchcock*, 175.

13 In the original script, as well as in the theatrical trailer, the sculptress who lives below Miss Torso is called "Miss Hearing Aid" by Jefferies. No mention of this is made in the film; in fact Jeff never speaks of her. The only remnant of this aspect of the script is found early in the film, when she fails to hear a neighbor greet her "Good morning," and has to be told again louder. For the purposes of this essay, I will refer to her as "Miss Hearing Aid," since the films gives her no other name.

14 There are several lines spoken, in the denouement, such as Miss Lonelyhearts's confession to the songwriter of the personal meaning for her of his songs, though Stella's line in the previous scene is the last dialogue that is presented in the foreground, and not a moment of "eavesdropping" on the neighbors.

15 Wallace Stevens, "Sunday Morning," in *The Collected Poems of Wallace Stevens*, ed. John N. Serio (New York: Vintage, 1990), 66.

Chapter 5

1 H. E. F. Donohue, "Remembrance of Murders Past: An Interview with Alfred Hitchcock," *The New York Times* (December 14, 1969).

2 From the opening monologue of "Death Sentence," *Alfred Hitchcock Presents*. Season 3, Episode 30, aired April 27, 1958.

3 Charlotte Chandler, *It's Only a Movie: Alfred Hitchcock, a Personal Biography* (New York: Simon & Schuster, 2005), 30.

4 Ibid., 32.

5 Ibid., 37.

6 Ibid., 33.

7 Donald Spoto, *The Dark Side of Genius: The Life of Alfred Hitchcock* (New York: Da Capo Press, 1983), 16.

8 Chandler, *It's Only a Movie*, 33.

9 Ibid., 34.

10 Ibid., 33.

11 Ibid.

12 Interview with Huw Wheldon. "Monitor." BBC, aired July 5, 1964.

13 This is a ubiquitous quotation attributed to Hitchcock, of unknown origin. No biography contains a mention of it.

14 Another frequent attribution to Hitchcock with an unknown source.

15 Laurent Bouzereau, *The Alfred Hitchcock Quote Book* (New York: Citadel Press, 1993), 166.

16 A ubiquitous Internet quotation, apparently taken from a news summary of quotations, December 31, 1963.

17 Patrick McGilligan, *Alfred Hitchcock: A Life in Darkness and Light* (New York: Reganbooks, 2003), 27.

18 Spoto, *Dark Side*, 107.

19 Ibid.

20 Interview with Oriana Fallaci, *Alfred Hitchcock: Interviews* (Jackson: University Press of Mississippi, 2003), 65.

21 McGilligan, *Darkness and* Light, 106. McGilligan lists *I Confess* as a Hitchcock film that portrays an ill-timed pregnancy, though it only existed in the script before Warner Brothers disallowed any mention of a child between Logan and Ruth.

22 I am not including children who are part of street or crowd scenes, simply part of the mise-en-scene.

23 Alfred Hitchcock, "The Enjoyment of Fear," *Good Housekeeping* 128 (February 1949): 39, 241–43.

24 While scholarship on the film is not plentiful, I do appreciate David Sterritt's excellent chapter on it in his *The Films of Alfred Hitchcock* (New York: Cambridge University Press, 1996), 74, in which he examines the film as Hitchcock's response to "the sociocultural ethos of the 1950s," and the masochistic position of 1950s conformity that plagues and deforms protagonist Manny Balestrero (Henry Fonda).

25 The film did not do well in the United States, though it was better received in Europe.

26 Quoted in "Guilt Trip: Hitchcock and *The Wrong Man*." Dir. Laurent Bouzereau, Blue Collar Productions, Warner Brothers, 2004.

27 Hitchcock shot a cameo appearance, where he stood in a diner as Henry Fonda sits down to a table to eat, but he did not use it, opting instead for the intro.

28 Of course, in *Spellbound*, John Ballantyne represses the memory of killing his brother, but their relationship is never explored.

29 Spoto, *Dark Side*, 114.

30 For a longer discussion of how milk functions in Hitchcock's films, see Chapter 3.

31 Sterritt, *Alfred Hitchcock*, 74. I think Sterritt actually means "of failing to perceive or acknowledge the decay of the middle class," since "failing to avoid a perception of decay" makes little sense (to me, at least), in the context of his argument.

32 Bouzereau, *Quote Book*, 181.

33 Barbara J. Buchanan, "Women Are a Nuisance," interview with Alfred Hitchcock, *Film Weekly* (September 20, 1935), 10. From *Hitchcock on Hitchcock*, ed. Sidney Gottlieb (Berkeley: University of California Press, 1995), 81.

Chapter 6

1 Lee Edelman, *No Future: Queer Theory and the Death Drive* (Durham: Duke University Press, 2004), 3.

2 Marilyn Wann, "Foreword: Fat Studies: An Invitation to Revolution," in *The Fat Studies Reader*, ed. Esther Rothblum and Sondra Solovay (New York: New York University Press, 2009), x.

3 Sander Gilman, *Fat Boys: A Slim Book* (Lincoln: University of Nebraska Press, 2004), 24–25.

4 Edelman, *No Future*, 11–12.

5 Michael Moon and Eve Kosofky Sedgwick, "Divinity: A Dossier, A Performance Piece, A Little-Understood Emotion," *Tendencies* (Durham: Duke University Press, 1994), 229–30.

6 Gilman, *Fat Boys*, 26.

7 For a fuller account of the Hitchcock/Hedren relationship, see Donald Spoto's 2010 *Spellbound by Beauty*.

8 Quite tellingly, Spoto does not mention Hedren's outburst in his *Spellbound by Beauty*, nor does he discredit or refute the account of Taylor which reports her insult. One wonders if Spoto was trying to avoid portraying Ms. Hedren as "difficult" or foul-mouthed.

9 Interview with Arthur Laurents, "*Rope* Unleashed," dir. Laurent Bouzereau, Universal Studios, 2000. When Laurents refers to the actors as "It," he referred to the homosexuality of Farley Granger and John Dall; he did not include James Stewart in that characterization.

10 Judith Butler, *Excitable Speech: A Politics of the Performative* (Berkeley: University of California Press, 1995).

11 Hitchcock never recovered from his former boss Michael Balcon's slight against him in the press, when he called him a "plump junior technician." Even thirty years later, Hitch shared with Charlotte Chandler, "it just hurt too much" to forgive and forget the insult.

12 Charlotte Chandler, *It's Only a Movie: Hitchcock, a Personal Biography* (New York: Simon & Schuster, 2005), 7.

13 One may dispute the characterization of these characters as "overtly" LGBT; I designate them as overt because most critics have agreed upon their queer identity, and within the films, they read more strongly than simple insinuation or overtures would permit.

14 Eve Sedgwick, "Queer and Now," *Tendencies* (Durham: Duke University Press, 1994), 8.

15 Ibid., 7–8.

16 Laura Mulvey, "Visual Pleasure and Narrative Cinema," *Screen* 16, no. 3 (1975): 6–18.

17 Laura Mulvey, "Afterthoughts on 'Visual Pleasure and Narrative Cinema,' Inspired by *Duel in the Sun*," *Framework* 15/16/17 (Summer 1981): 12–15.

18 Rob Horning, "Precarity and 'affective resistance'," *The New Inquiry* (February 14, 2012). http://thenewinquiry.com/blogs/marginal-utility/precarity-and-affective-resistance/.

19 Laurent Bouzereau, *The Alfred Hitchcock Quote Book* (New York: A Citadel Press Book, 1993), 185.

20 Francois Truffaut, ed., *Hitchcock* (New York: Simon & Schuster, 1984).

21 Bouzereau, *Quote Book*, 167.

22 Interview with Eva Marie Saint, *Destination Hitchcock: The Making of North by Northwest*. Dir. Laurent Bouzereau, 2000.

23 Chandler, *It's Only*, 166.

24 "A Talk with Hitchcock." *Telescope*. Hosted and produced by Fletcher Markle, January 1, 1964.

Enhanced Filmography

1) *The Pleasure Garden* (1925)

Screenplay: Eliot Stannard, based on the novel *The Pleasure Garden* by Oliver Sandys

Producer: Michael Balcon, Erich Pommer, Bavaria Film, Gainsborough Pictures, Münchner Lichtspielkunst AG (Emelka)

Runtime: 75 minutes

Cast: Virginia Valli, Carmelita Geraghty, Miles Mander, John Stuart, Ferdinand Martini, Florence Helminger

During two intercut dinner table sequences, two couples sit with tea sets and small plates in front of them; the couple that is eating and drinking end up falling in love.

2) *The Lodger* (also titled *The Lodger: A Story of the London Fog*) (1927)

Screenplay: Eliot Stannard, Alfred Hitchcock (uncredited), based on the novel *The Lodger* and the play *Who Is He?*, both by Marie Belloc Lowndes

Producer: Gainsborough Pictures, Carlyle Blackwell Productions, Michael Balcon, Carlyle Blackwell

Runtime: 68 minutes

Cast: Marie Ault, Arthur Chesney, June, Malcolm Keen, Ivor Novello

When the Lodger (Ivor Novello) arrives at the Buntings' boardinghouse, he immediately requests some bread, butter, and a glass of milk. Hitchcock wanted to suggest that he was preserving his waifish figure.

3) *Downhill* (*When Boys Leave Home*) (1927)

Screenplay: Constance Collier (play), Ivor Novello (play), Eliot Stannard (adaptation)

Producer: Gainsborough Pictures, Michael Balcon, C. M. Woolf

Runtime: 74 minutes

Roddy and his best friend Tim meet Mabel at the sweets shop where she works. After rejecting Mabel's advances, Roddy attempts to help a customer while she kisses Tim in a back room. He sells an expensive box of chocolates to a little boy who does not have enough money. This backfires when the boy returns with all his friends, looking to buy more boxes with their own meager coin.

4) *The Ring* (1927)

Screenplay: Alfred Hitchcock, Alma Reville (uncredited), Eliot Stannard (uncredited)

Producer: British International Pictures, John Maxwell

Runtime: 72 minutes

Cast: Carl Brisson, Lillian Hall-Davis, Ian Hunter, Forrester Harvey, Harry Terry, Gordon Harker

Jack (Carl Brisson) wins the most important match of his career, and he and his entourage return to his flat to celebrate with Jack's wife. "We'll toast . . . but not drink until my wife gets here." A glass of champagne is shown going completely flat to indicate the passing of time, and hint at his wife's affair.

5) *The Farmer's Wife* (1928)

Screenplay: Eliot Stannard, Leslie Arliss (uncredited), Alfred Hitchcock (uncredited), J. E. Hunter (uncredited), Norman Lee (uncredited), based on the play *The Farmer's Wife* by Eden Phillpotts

Producer: British International Pictures

Runtime: 129 minutes

Cast: Jameson Thomas, Lillian Hall-Davis, Gordon Harker, Gibb McLaughlin, Maud Gill, Louie Pounds

Before Mr. Sweetland's disastrous attempt at courting three eligible bachelorettes around town, his servant (Gordon Harker) remarks cryptically (though drunkenly), "Beer drinking don't do half the harm of love-making."

6) *Easy Virtue* (1928)

Screenplay: Eliot Stannard, based on the play *Easy Virtue* by Noël Coward

Producer: Gainsborough Pictures, Michael Balcon

Runtime: 70 minutes

Cast: Isabel Jeans, Franklin Dyall, Eric Bransby Williams, Ian Hunter, Robin Irvine, Violet Farebrother

A decanter of brandy is used as the main piece of evidence in the divorce case against the perfectly innocent Larita; the following scene shows that it belongs to her drunkard husband.

7) *Champagne* (1928)

Screenplay: Alfred Hitchcock, Eliot Stannard, based on the novel *Champagne* by Walter C. Mycroft

Producer: John Maxwell, British International Pictures

Runtime: 86 minutes

Cast: Betty Balfour, Jean Bradin, Ferdinand von Alten, Gordon Harker

A spoiled heiress goes from making cocktails at swanky parties to trying to bake for herself and her father after he tells her that their champagne empire fortune has been lost. The hard biscuits and poor cooking serve as reminders of how naïve and unskilled the heiress truly is.

8) *The Manxman* (1929)

Screenplay: Eliot Stannard, based on the novel *The Manxman* by Sir Hall Caine

Producer: British International Pictures, John Maxwell

Runtime: 110 minutes

Cast: Carl Brisson, Malcolm Keen, Anny Ondra, Randle Ayrton, Clare Greet

Pete arrives home and sees only one place setting on the table where two usually set; next to the plate, Kate has left her wedding ring and a goodbye note, telling him that she loves another man.

9) *Blackmail* (1929)

Screenplay: Alfred Hitchcock, Benn W. Levy, Michael Powell (uncredited), based on the play *Blackmail* by Charles Bennett

Producer: British International Pictures, John Maxwell

Runtime: 85 minutes

Cast: Anny Ondra, Sara Allgood, Charles Paton, John Longden, Donald Calthrop, Cyril Ritchard, Joan Barry (voice, uncredited)

As our heroine Alice, who has just stabbed a man to death in self-defense, is about to slice open a fresh loaf of bread at the lunch table, the

incriminating word "knife," repeated by a lunch companion, resounds in her head, climaxing as she hurls the bread knife across the room.

10) *Murder!* (1930)

Screenplay: Alfred Hitchcock, Walter C. Mycroft, Alma Reville, based on the novel and play *Enter Sir John* by Clemence Dane and Helen Simpson

Producer: British International Pictures, John Maxwell

Runtime: 92 minutes

Cast: Herbert Marshall, Norah Baring, Phyllis Konstam, Edward Chapman, Miles Mander, Esme Percy

Sir John Menier (Herbert Marshall) surmises that circus performer Handel Fane (Esme Percy) was present at the scene of Edna Druce's murder when he spies a bottle of Martell brandy in his dressing room; a brandy decanter had been mysteriously emptied at the scene of the crime.

11) *The Skin Game* (1931)

Screenplay: Alfred Hitchcock, Alma Reville, based on the play *The Skin Game* by John Galsworthy

Producer: British International Pictures, John Maxwell

Runtime: 77 minutes

Cast: C. V. France, Helen Haye, Jill Esmond, Edmund Gwenn, John Longden, Phyllis Konstam

In the first scene of the film, the children of the two feuding families meet on a road, the upper class girl on horseback and the nouveau riche boy in a convertible car. While implying that her family would like to maintain a certain sense of class, Jill eats an apple and speaks with a full mouth.

12) *Rich and Strange* (also titled *East of Shanghai*) (1931)

Screenplay: Alfred Hitchcock, Alma Reville, Val Valentine, based on the novel *East of Shanghai* by Dale Collins

Producer: John Maxwell, British International Pictures,

Runtime: 83 minutes

Cast: Henry Kendall, Joan Barry, Percy Marmont, Betty Amann, Elsie Randolph

Married world travelers Fred and Emily Hill (Henry Kendall and Joan Barry) promptly vomit over the side of a Chinese junk when they realize that they have just been served cat meat.

13) *Number 17* (1932)

Screenplay: Rodney Ackland, Alfred Hitchcock, Alma Reville, based on the play *Number Seventeen* by Joseph Jefferson Farjeon

Producer: Leon M. Lion, British International Pictures, John Maxwell

Runtime: 63 minutes

Cast: Leon M. Lion, Anne Grey, John Stuart, Donald Calthrop, Barry Jones, Ann Casson

Chasing the diamond necklace thieves onto a moving train, the drunken tramp Ben (Leon M. Lion) stumbles into a car filled with cases of EMU brand "tonic wine." A few minutes later, we see Ben imbibing merrily and holding the missing necklace that the rest of the characters are scrambling for.

14) *Waltzes from Vienna* (also titled *Strauss' Great Waltz*) (1934)

Screenplay: Heinz Reichert and Ernst Marischka

Producer: Thomas Charles Arnold, Gaumont British Picture Corporation, Tom Arnold Films

Runtime: 80 minutes

Cast: Jessie Matthews, Edmund Gwenn, Fay Compton, Esmond Knight, Frank Vosper, Robert Hale

While trying to convince her love, Johan Strauss, Jr. to work in her father's bakery so she can marry him, Resi regales him with tales of the famous historical patrons of the shop. She proudly points to a coffee stain on the wall that resulted from a cup being hurled at General Radetzky by a famous painter.

15) *The Man Who Knew Too Much* (1934)

Screenplay: Charles Bennett, Edwin Greenwood, A. R. Rawlinson, Emlyn Williams, D. B. Wyndham-Lewis

Producer: Ivor Montagu, Gaumont British Picture Corporation, Michael Balcon

Runtime: 75 minutes

Cast: Leslie Banks, Edna Best, Peter Lorre, Frank Vosper, Hugh Wakefield, Nova Pilbeam

The leader of the assassins forces Mrs. Brockett to stay and serve them food and drinks, and to humiliate her, makes her work in only undergarments. One member of the group appears to pinch her bottom, but was only reaching for an hors d'oeuvre behind her.

16) *The 39 Steps* (1935)

Screenplay: Charles Bennett, Ian Hay, based on the novel *The 39 Steps* by John Buchan

Producer: Gaumont British Picture Corporation, Michael Balcon, Ivor Montagu

Runtime: 86 minutes

Cast: Robert Donat, Madeleine Carroll, Lucie Mannheim, Godfrey Tearle, Dame Peggy Ashcroft, John Laurie

When spy Annabella Smith (Lucie Mannheim) seeks sanctuary in Richard Hannay's (Robert Donat) apartment, he serves her cold fish and crusty bread.

17) *Secret Agent* (1936)

Screenplay: Charles Bennett, Ian Hay, Jesse Lasky Jr., Alma Reville, based on the play *Secret Agent* by Campbell Dixon and the novel *Ashenden* by W. Somerset Maugham

Producer: Gaumont British Picture Corporation, Michael Balcon, Ivor Montagu

Runtime: 86 minutes

Cast: John Gielgud, Peter Lorre, Madeleine Carroll, Robert Young, Percy Marmont, Florence Kahn

When British officer Ashenden (John Gielgud) resigns his intelligence post, he leaves the note: "Now that I have resigned, if you want a successor for me, I can give you the name of a good, reliable butcher."

18) *Sabotage* (1936)

Screenplay: Charles Bennett, E. V. H. Emmett, Ian Hay, Alma Reville, Helen Simpson, based on the novel *Secret Agent* by Joseph Conrad

Producer: Gaumont British Picture Corporation, Michael Balcon, Ivor Montagu

Runtime: 76 minutes

Cast: Sylvia Sidney, Oskar Homolka, Desmond Tester, John Loder, Joyce Barbour, Matthew Boulton

Ted (John Loder) blanches when Mrs. Verloc (Sylvia Sydney) tries to order her brother a poached egg: "A poached egg?! The roast beef would turn over in its gravy!"

19) *Young and Innocent* (also titled *The Girl Was Young*) (1937)

Screenplay: Anthony Armstrong, Charles Bennett, Edwin Greenwood, Alma Reville, Gerald Savory, based on the novel *A Shilling for Candles* by Josephine Tey

Producer: Gaumont British Picture Corporation, Edward Black

Runtime: 83 minutes

Cast: Nova Pilbeam, Derrick De Marney, Percy Marmont, Edward Rigby, Mary Clare, John Longden

Erica Burgoyne's (Nova Pilbeam) younger brothers agree that a murderer on the run should take a stash of chocolate with him.

20) *The Lady Vanishes* (1938)

Screenplay: Sidney Gilliat, Frank Launder, based on the story "The Wheel Spins" by Ethel Lina White

Producer: Gainsborough Pictures, Edward Black

Runtime: 96 minutes

Cast: Margaret Lockwood, Michael Redgrave, Paul Lukas, Damn May Whitty, Cecil Parker, Linden Travers

It takes the discovery of a discarded teabag—of *Harriman's Herbal Tea,* to be precise ("A Million Mexicans Drink It!" on the box)—to convince Gilbert (Michael Redgrave) that Iris (Margaret Lockwood) was not hallucinating the presence of Miss Froy on their train to London.

21) *Jamaica Inn* (1939)

Screenplay: Sidney Gilliat, Joan Harrison, J. B. Preistley, Alma Reville, based on the novel *Jamaica Inn* by Daphne Du Maurier

Producer: Erich Pommer, Mayflower Pictures Corporation, Charles Laughton

Runtime: 98 minutes

Cast: Charles Laughton, Horace Hodges, Maureen O'Hara, Hay Petrie, Frederick Piper, Emlyn Williams

Sir Humphrey, who is in on the wrongdoing, makes light of the smugglers at Jamaica Inn in front of his colleagues. "Got any good brandies in?" one jokes. "Why yes," responds Trehearne, producing a "list" and showing it only to Humphrey; the list is actually proof that Trehearne is an undercover police officer.

22) *Rebecca* (1940)

Screenplay: Joan Harrison, Michael Hogan, Phillip MacDonald, Robert E. Sherwood, based on the novel *Rebecca* by Daphne Du Maurier

Producer: David O. Selznick, Selznick International Pictures

Runtime: 130 minutes

Cast: Laurence Olivier, Joan Fontaine, George Sanders, Judith Anderson, Nigel Bruce, Reginald Denny

The unnamed protagonist (Joan Fontaine) begins the film a wispy child who picks at scrambled eggs, and throughout the film, matures into a strong woman who packs a picnic of chicken, baguette, and a magnum of champagne for her and her husband Maxim (Laurence Olivier).

23) *Foreign Correspondent* (1940)

Screenplay: Robert Benchley, Charles Bennett, Joan Harrison, James Hilton, Ben Hecht (uncredited)

Producer: Walter Wanger Productions

Runtime: 120 minutes

Cast: Joel McCrea, Laraine Day, Herbert Marshall, George Sanders, Albert Bassermann, Robert Benchley

Johnny Jones (Joel McCrea) awkwardly tries to communicate with a foreign ambassador, first in English, then French, then German; the situation is resolved when a waiter passes by, and the "universal language" of champagne is spoken.

24) *Mr. & Mrs. Smith* (1941)

Screenplay: Norman Krasna

Producer: Harry E. Edington, RKO Radio Pictures

Runtime: 95 minutes

Cast: Carole Lombard, Robert Montgomery, Gene Raymond, Jack Carson, Philip Merivale, Lucile Watson

David Smith agrees to a double blind date at the Florida Club to make his wife jealous. Both women turn out to be low-class: one struggles with her pheasant, and the other laments not having ordered chop suey.

25) *Suspicion* (1941)

Screenplay: Samson Raphaelson, Joan Harrison, Alma Reville, based on the novel *Before the Fact* by Anthony Berkeley

Producer: Harry E. Edington, RKO Radio Pictures

Runtime: 99 minutes

Cast: Cary Grant, Joan Fontaine, Cedric Hardwicke, Nigel Bruce, Dame May Whitty, Isabel Jeans, Auriol Lee, Leo G. Carroll

After kissing Johnnie Aysgarth (Cary Grant) for the first time, Lina (Joan Fontaine) bounds into the dining room, and promptly asks the butler for roast beef, "well done," as her parents quibble over the freshness of the horseradish.

26) *Saboteur* (1942)

Screenplay: Joan Harrison, Dorothy Parker, Peter Viertel, Alfred Hitchcock (uncredited)

Producer: Jack H. Skirball, Frank Lloyd Productions, Universal Pictures, Frank Lloyd

Runtime: 109 minutes

Cast: Priscilla Lane, Robert Cummings, Otto Kruger, Alan Baxter, Clem Bevans, Norman Lloyd

A corrupt police office feeds Pat (Priscilla Lane) milk and sandwiches (the same meal Norman Bates serves Marion) before handing her over to the movie's villain Tobin (Otto Kruger).

27) *Shadow of a Doubt* (1943)

Screenplay: Sally Benson, Alma Reville, Thornton Wilder, based on an original story by Gordon McDonell

Producer: Jack H. Skirball, Skirball Productions, Universal Pictures

Runtime: 108 minutes

Cast: Teresa Wright, Joseph Cotten, Macdonald Carey, Henry Travers, Patricia Collinge, Hume Cronyn

Herb (Hume Cronyn) threatens to slip poisonous mushrooms among the regular ones that Joe Newton (Henry Travers) eats on top of steak "when the meat isn't very good."

28) *Lifeboat* (1944)

Screenplay: Jo Swerling, Ben Hecht (uncredited), Alfred Hitchcock (uncredited), original story by John Steinbeck

Producer: Alfred Hitchcock, Kenneth Macgowan, Twentieth Century Fox Film Corporation, William Goetz, Darryl F. Zanuck

Runtime: 97 minutes

Cast: Tallulah Bankhead, William Bendix, Walter Slezak, Mary Anderson, John Hodiak, Henry Hull, Hume Cronyn

When a German supply ship hails the stranded lifeboat, Connie Porter (Tallulah Bankhead) facetiously translates their hello: "He says yes, they

have coffee . . . and wiener schnitzel and pigs' knuckles and sauerkraut and apple strudel . . ."

29) *Bon Voyage* (1944)

Screenplay: Angus MacPhail, J. O. C. Orton

Producer: Ministry of Information

Runtime: 34 minutes

Cast: John Blythe

Royal Air Force Sergeant John Dougall is aided by French Resistance allies who provide him and his POW friend with bicycles and a crust of bread attached.

30) *Aventure Malgache* (1944)

Screenplay: Jules Francois Clermont

Producer: Ministry of Information

Runtime: 32 minutes

Cast: Paul Bonifas, Paul Clarus, Jean Dattas, Andre Frere, Guy Le Feuvre, Paulette Preney

When Paul (Paul Clarus) refuses to swear allegiance to the Vichy French, corrupt chief of police Michel (Paul Bonifas) spits a shot of rum in his face.

31) *Spellbound* (1945)

Screenplay: Ben Hecht, Angus MacPhail, May E. Romm (uncredited), based on the novel *The House of Dr. Edwardes* by Frances Beeding, John Palmer (uncredited), Hilary St. George Sanders (uncredited)

Producer: David O. Selznick, Selznick International Pictures, Vanguard Films

Runtime: 111 minutes

Cast: Ingrid Bergman, Gregory Peck, Michael Chekhov, Leo G. Carroll, Rhonda Fleming, John Emery

John Ballantyne, posing as Dr. Edwardes (Gregory Peck) offers Constance Petersen (Ingrid Bergman) a choice of ham or liverwurst sandwich on an impromptu picnic—their first date. She happily chooses liverwurst, the more decadent option.

32) *Notorious* (1946)

Screenplay: Ben Hecht, Alfred Hitchcock (uncredited), based on the story "The Song of the Dragon" by John Taintor Foote

Producer: Vanguard Films, RKO Radio Pictures, Alfred Hitchcock

Runtime: 101 minutes

Cast: Cary Grant, Ingrid Bergman, Claude Rains, Louis Calhern, Leopoldine Konstantin, Reinhold Schünzel

In the original three drafts of the script, Alicia (Ingrid Bergman) is shown slaving away in a kitchen to make Devlin (Cary Grant) *arroz con pollo*, with sugared grapefruit for dessert. This scene was abandoned, and the chicken is only talked about.

33) *The Paradine Case* (1947)

Screenplay: Alma Reville, David O. Selznick, James Bridie (uncredited), Ben Hecht (uncredited), based on the novel *The Paradine Case* by Robert Hichens

Producer: Vanguard Films, Selznick Studio, David O. Selznick

Runtime: 125 minutes

Cast: Gregory Peck, Ann Todd, Charles Laughton, Charles Coburn, Ethel Barrymore, Louis Jourdan, Valli

During the trial of Maddalena Paradine, the prosecutor reads the contents of the poisoned Captain's last meal: roast chicken, roasted potatoes, cauliflower au gratin, and a single glass of burgundy.

34) *Rope* (1948)

Screenplay: Hume Cronyn, Arthur Laurents, Ben Hecht (uncredited), based on the play *Rope* by Patrick Hamilton

Producer: Warner Bros., Transatlantic Pictures, Sidney Bernstein, Alfred Hitchcock

Runtime: 80 minutes

Cast: Dick Hogan, John Dall, Farley Granger, Edith Evanson, Douglas Dick, Joan Chandler, Constance Collier, Cedric Hardwicke

Housekeeper Mrs. Wilson reports she went to five different delis to find the right pâté for Philip and Brandon's party.

35) *Under Capricorn* (1949)

Screenplay: James Bridie, Hume Cronyn, Peter Ustinov (uncredited), Joseph Shearing (uncredited), based on the play *Under Capricorn* by John Colton and Margaret Linden, and the novel *Under Capricorn* by Helen Simpson

Producer: Transatlantic Pictures, Sidney Bernstein, Alfred Hitchcock

Runtime: 117 minutes

Cast: Ingrid Bergman, Joseph Cotten, Michael Wilding, Margaret Leighton, Cecil Parker, Denis O'Dea

When Sam Flusky throws a dinner party (one which contains conspicuously no wives, who fear for their reputations), he puts out relish trays of oranges, olives, carrots, and grapes.

36) *Stage Fright* (1950)

Screenplay: Whitfield Cook, Alma Reville, James Bridie (uncredited), Ranald MacDougall (uncredited), based on the novel *Man Running* by Selwyn Jepson

Producer: Warner Bros., Alfred Hitchcock

Runtime: 110 minutes

Cast: Jane Wyman, Marlene Dietrich, Michael Wilding, Richard Todd, Alastair Sim, Sybil Thorndike

The blackmailing Nellie Goode has a signature drink: "Gin and lemon. Easy on the lemon."

37) *Strangers on a Train* (1951)

Screenplay: Raymond Chandler, Whitfield Cook, Czenzi Ormonde, Ben Hecht (uncredited), based on the novel *Strangers on a Train* by Patricia Highsmith

Producer: Warner Bros., Alfred Hitchcock

Runtime: 110 minutes

Cast: Farley Granger, Ruth Roman, Robert Walker, Leo G. Carroll, Patricia Hitchcock, Kasey Rogers

At the fair, shortly before she is murdered, Miriam craves hot dogs, ice cream, popcorn, and Bruno's attentions.

38) *I Confess* (1953)

Screenplay: William Archibald, George Tabori, based on the play *Nos deus consciences (Our Two Consciences)* by Paul Anthelme

Producer: Warner Bros., Sidney Bernstein, Alfred Hitchcock

Runtime: 95 minutes

Cast: Montgomery Clift, Anne Baxter, Karl Malden, Brian Aherne, O. E. Hasse, Roger Dann

On the set, Montgomery Clift often carried around a pitcher of vodka and painkillers; as a result, several of his scenes reveal a glassy-eyed Father Logan.

39) *Dial M for Murder* (1954)

Screenplay: Frederick Knott, adapted from his own play *Dial M for Murder*

Producer: Warner Bros., Alfred Hitchcock

Runtime: 105 minutes

Cast: Ray Milland, Grace Kelly, Robert Cummings, John Williams, Anthony Dawson, Leo Britt

Tony Wendice (Ray Milland) watches his wife Margot (Grace Kelly) and Mark Halliday (Robert Cummings) quietly making pasta together, and discerns right away that they are in love.

40) *Rear Window* (1954)

Screenplay: John Michael Hayes, based on the short story "It Had to be Murder"

Producer: Paramount Pictures, Patron Inc., Alfred Hitchcock

Runtime: 112 minutes

Cast: James Stewart, Grace Kelly, Wendell Corey, Thelma Ritter, Raymond Burr, Judith Evelyn

Because Jeff (James Stewart) is unable to leave his apartment due to a broken leg, Lisa Freemont (Grace Kelly) brings lobster and frites from the 21 Club to his apartment.

41) *To Catch a Thief* (1955)

Screenplay: John Michael Hayes, Alec Coppel (uncredited), based the novel *To Catch a Thief* by David Dodge

Producer: Alfred Hitchcock, Paramount Pictures

Runtime: 106 minutes

Cast: Cary Grant, Grace Kelly, Jessie Royce Landis, John Williams, Charles Vanel, Brigitte Auber

On a picnic in the south of France, Francey (Grace Kelly) pulls chicken from her basket and provocatively asks John Robie (Cary Grant), "You want a breast or a leg?"

42) *The Trouble with Harry* (1955)

Screenplay: John Michael Hayes, based on the novel *The Trouble with Harry* by Jack Trevor Story

Producer: Herbert Coleman, Alfred J. Hitchcock Productions, Paramount Pictures, Alfred Hitchcock

Runtime: 99 minutes

Cast: Edmund Gwenn, John Forsythe, Mildred Natwick, Mildred Dunnock, Jerry Mathers, Royal Dano

When Captain Albert finds that, instead of shooting Harry, he has actually killed a hare, he proposes that they make a rabbit stew.

43) *The Man Who Knew Too Much* (1956)

Screenplay: John Michael Hayes, Angus MacPhail (uncredited), based on a story by Charles Bennett, D. B. Wyndham-Lewis

Producer: Herbert Coleman, Paramount Pictures, Filwite Productions, Alfred Hitchcock

Runtime: 120 minutes

Cast: James Stewart, Doris Day, Brenda de Banzie, Bernard Miles, Ralph Truman, Daniel Gélin

The McKennas (James Stewart and Doris Day) embarrass themselves in a Moroccan restaurant through their difficulties in grabbing roast chicken with their injera bread.

44) *The Wrong Man* (1956)

Screenplay: Maxwell Anderson, Angus MacPhail

Producer: Herbert Coleman, Warner Bros., Alfred Hitchcock

Runtime: 105 minutes

Cast: Henry Fonda, Vera Miles, Anthony Quayle, Harold J. Stone, Charles Cooper, John Heldabrand

When Manny (Henry Fonda) is released from prison, his wife Rose (Vera Miles) comforts him with the promise of coffee and lasagna at home.

45) *Vertigo* (1958)

Screenplay: Alec Coppel, Samuel A. Taylor, Maxwell Anderson (uncredited), based on the novel *D'Entre Les Morts* by Pierre Boileau and Thomas Narcejac

Producer: Herbert Coleman, Paramount Pictures, Alfred J. Hitchcock Productions, Alfred Hitchcock

Runtime: 128 minutes

Cast: James Stewart, Kim Novak, Barbara Bel Geddes, Tom Helmore, Henry Jones, Raymond Bailey

After making love, Judy Barton (Kim Novak) declares her hunger for "one of [Ernie's] beautiful steaks."

46) *North by Northwest* (1959)

Screenplay: Ernest Lehman

Producer: Herbert Coleman, Metro-Goldwyn-Mayer (MGM), Alfred Hitchcock

Runtime: 136 minutes

Cast: Cary Grant, Eva Marie Saint, James Mason, Jessie Royce Landis, Leo G. Carroll, Josephine Hutchinson

Before she seduces Roger Thornhill (Cary Grant), double agent Eve Kendall (Eva Marie Saint) recommends he try the brook trout: "a little trouty, but good."

47) *Psycho* (1960)

Screenplay: Joseph Stefano, based on the novel *Psycho* by Robert Bloch

Producer: Shamley Productions, Alfred Hitchcock

Runtime: 109 minutes

Cast: Anthony Perkins, Vera Miles, John Gavin, Janet Leigh, Martin Balsam, John McIntire

Because the film was shot in black and white, Hitchcock chose to use Bosco chocolate syrup for the blood in the shower scene. It was Anthony Perkins's idea to have Norman Bates munch on candy corn throughout the film.

48) *The Birds* (1963)

Screenplay: Evan Hunter, based on the short story "The Birds" by Daphne Du Maurier

Producer: Universal Pictures, Alfred J. Hitchcock Productions, Alfred Hitchcock

Runtime: 119 minutes

Cast: Tippi Hedren, Suzanne Pleshette, Rod Taylor, Jessica Tandy, Veronica Cartwright, Ethel Griffies

At the Tides Restaurant, ornithologist Mrs. Bundy (Ethel Griffies) explains that birds are peaceful creatures; she is interrupts by a waitress barking an order for "Fried chicken!"

49) *Marnie* (1964)

Screenplay: Jay Presson Allen, based on the novel *Marnie* by Winston Graham

Producer: Universal Pictures, Alfred J. Hitchcock Productions, Alfred Hitchcock

Runtime: 130 minutes

Cast: Tippi Hedren, Sean Connery, Diane Baker, Martin Gabel, Louise Latham, Bob Sweeney

Marnie (Tippi Hedren) is jealous that her mother (Louise Latham) is baking a pecan pie for neighbor girl Jesse, whom she considers a rival for her affections.

50) *Torn Curtain* (1966)

Screenplay: Brian Moore, Willis Hall (uncredited), Keith Waterhouse (uncredited)

Producer: Universal Pictures, Alfred Hitchcock

Runtime: 128 minutes

Cast: Paul Newman, Julie Andrews, Lila Kedrova, Hansjörg Felmy, Tamara Toumanova, Wolfgang Keiling

Countess Kuchinska (Lila Kedrova) seeks sponsorship to get to America so that she can stop drinking German coffee and smoking Russian cigarettes.

51) *Topaz* (1969)

Screenplay: Samuel A. Taylor, based on the novel *Topaz* by Leon Uris

Producer: Herbert Coleman, Universal Pictures, Alfred Hitchcock

Runtime: 143 minutes

Cast: Frederick Stafford, Dany Robin, John Vernon, Karin Dor, Michel Piccoli, Philippe Noiret

Cuban spies working against Castro have placed surveillance cameras in interesting places, including large Cuban sandwiches and chicken carcasses.

52) *Frenzy* (1972)

Screenplay: Anthony Shaffer, based on the novel *Goodbye Piccadilly, Farewell Leicester Square* by Arthur La Bern

Producer: William Hill, Alfred Hitchcock, Universal Pictures

Runtime: 116 minutes

Cast: Jon Finch, Alec McCowen, Barry Foster, Billie Whitelaw, Anna Massey, Barbara Leigh-Hunt

After Bob Rusk (Barry Foster) rapes and kills Brenda Blaney (Barbara Leigh-Hunt), he resumes eating the apple she had packed for her "frugal" lunch.

53) *Family Plot* (1976)

Screenplay: Ernest Lehman, based on the novel *The Rainbird Pattern* by Victor Canning

Producer: Universal Pictures, Alfred Hitchcock

Runtime: 120 minutes

Cast: Karen Black, Bruce Dern, Barbara Harris, William Devane, Ed Lauter, Cathleen Nesbitt

Kidnapper Fran (Karen Black) frets that her victim did not finish his wine, reasoning that it was because she had overcooked his veal parmesan.

Bibliography

Bakhtin, Mikhael. *Rabelais and His World.* Bloomington: Indiana University Press, 1965.

Balcon, Michael. *London Sunday Dispatch.* August 25, 1940.

Barton, Sabrina. "CrissCross: Paranoia and Projection in *Strangers on a Train.*" In *Out in Culture: Gay, Lesbian and Queer Essays in Popular Culture,* edited by Corey K. Creekmur and Alexander Doty, 216–38. Durham: Duke University Press, 1995.

Bouzereau, Laurent. *Destination Hitchcock: The Making of North By Northwest.* Berkeley: Universal Studios, 1990.

Bouzereau, Laurent. *The Alfred Hitchcock Quote Book.* New York: Citadel Press, 1993.

Bouzereau, Laurent. "*Rope* Unleashed." Interview with Arthur Laurents. Universal Studios, 2000.

Bouzereau, Laurent, Dir. *Guilt Trip: Hitchcock and The Wrong Man.* Berkeley: Blue Collar Productions, Warner Bros., 2004.

Bouzereau, Laurent. *Hitchcock Piece by Piece.* New York: ABRAMS, 2010.

Braziel, Jana Evans and Kathleen LeBesco. *Bodies Out of Bounds.* Berkeley: University of California Press, 2001.

Buchanan, Barbara J. "Women Are a Nuisance." *Film Weekly.* September 20, 1935.

Butler, Judith. *Excitable Speech: A Politics of the Performative.* Berkeley: University of California Press, 1995.

Chandler, Charlotte. *It's Only a Movie: Hitchcock, a Personal Biography.* New York: Simon & Schuster, 2005.

Christ, Ronald. "*Strangers on a Train: The Pattern of Encounter.*" *Focus on Culture.* Edited by Albert LaValley. New York: Prentice Hall, 1972.

Coffin, Lesley L. *Hitchcock's Stars: Alfred Hitchcock and the Hollywood Studio System.* Lanham: Rowan & Littlefield, 2014.

De Rosa, Steven. *Writing with Hitchcock: The Collaboration of Alfred Hitchcock and John Michael Hayes.* New York and London: Faber and Faber, 2001.

Deutelbaum, Marshall and Leland Poague. *A Hitchcock Reader.* Hoboken: Wiley-Blackwell, 2009.

Donohue, H. E. F. "Remembrance of Murders Past: An Interview with Alfred Hitchcock." *The New York Times.* December 14, 1969.

Douchet, Jean. "Hitch et Son Public." *Cahiers du Cinema* 19, no. 3 (1960): 10.

Edelman, Lee. *No Future: Queer Theory and the Death Drive.* Durham: Duke University Press, 2004.

Fallacci, Oriana. *Alfred Hitchcock: Interviews.* Jackson: University of Mississippi Press, 2003.

Freedman, Jonathan and Richard Millington, eds. *Alfred Hitchcock's America*. Oxford: Oxford University Press, 1999.

Gilman, Sander. *Fat Boys*. Lincoln: University of Nebraska Press, 2004.

Gottlieb, Sidney, ed. *Hitchcock on Hitchcock*. Berkeley: University of California Press, 1995.

Hitchcock, Alfred. "Hitchcock Responds to 'Deserter Charge'." *New York World-Telegram*. August 27, 1940.

Hitchcock, Alfred. "The Woman Who Knows Too Much." *McCall's*. (March, 1956): 12–14.

Hitchcock, Alfred. *Hitchcock on Hitchcock: Selected Writings and Interviews*. Edited by Sidney Gottlieb. Berkeley: University of California Press, 1997.

Hitchcock, Alfred. *Hitchcock on Hitchcock Volume Two: Selected Writings and Interviews*. Edited by Sidney Gottlieb. Berkeley: University of California Press, 2014.

Horning, Rob. "Precarity and Affective Resistance." *The New Inquiry*. February 14, 2012. http://thenewinquiry.com/blogs/marginal-utility/precarity-and-affective-resistance/.

Hurston, Zora Neale. *Their Eyes Were Watching God*. New York: J. B. Lippincott, Inc., 1937.

Johnston, Alva. "300 Pound Prophet Comes to Hollywood." *Saturday Evening Post* 215, no. 47 (May 22, 1943): 12.

Kapsis, Robert E. *Hitchcock: The Making of a Reputation*. Chicago: University of Chicago Press, 1990.

Leff, Leonard J. *Hitchcock and Selznick: The Rich and Strange Collaboration of Alfred Hitchcock and David O. Selznick*. New York: Grove Press, 1988.

Leitch, Thomas and Leland Poague. *A Companion to Alfred Hitchcock*. Hoboken: Wiley-Blackwell, 2014.

Lewis, Jon. *Essential Cinema: An Introduction to Film Analysis*. Boston: Wadsworth, 2014.

Markle, Fletcher. "A Talk With Hitchcock." *Telescope*. CBC Television. January 1, 1964.

McGilligan, Patrick. *Alfred Hitchcock: A Life in Darkness and Light*. New York: Regan/Harper Collins, 2003.

Modleski, Tania. *The Women Who Knew Too Much: Hitchcock and Feminist Theory*. New York: Routledge, 2005.

Mogg, Ken. *The Alfred Hitchcock Story*. London: Titan Books, 2008.

Moon, Michael and Eve Kosofsky Sedgwick. "Divinity: A Dossier, A performance Piece, A Little-Understood Emotion." In *Tendencies*. Durham: Duke University Press, 1994, 215–52.

Mulvey, Laura. "Visual Pleasure and Narrative Cinema." *Screen* 16, no. 3. (Spring 1975): 6–18.

Mulvey, Laura. "Afterthoughts on 'Visual Pleasure and Narrative Cinema, Inspired by *Duel in the Sun*.'" *Framework* 15/16/17, Summer 1981.

O'Connell, Pat Hitchcock and Laurent Bouzereau. *Alma Hitchcock: The Woman Behind the Man*. New York: Berkley Books, 2003.

Olsson, Jan. *Hitchcock a la Carte*. Durham: Duke University Press, 2015.

Rebello, Stephen. *Alfred Hitchcock and the Making of Psycho*. New York: St. Martins, Griffin, 1990.

Roberts, Katharine. "Mystery Man: Thrills and Chills of Alfred Hitchcock." *Collier's Weekly.* (August 5, 1939): 22.
Rothblum, Esther and Sondra Solovay, eds. *The Fat Studies Reader.* New York: New York University Press, 2009.
Rothman, William. *Hitchcock: The Murderous Gaze.* Cambridge, MA: Harvard University Press, 1982.
Ryall, Tom. *Alfred Hitchcock & the British Cinema.* Urbana: University of Illinois Press, 1986.
Sedgwick, Eve Kosofsky. "Queer and Now." In *Tendencies.* Durham: Duke University Press, 1994, 1–22.
Selznick, David O. Archive, *The Harry Ransom Center.* Austin: University of Texas at Austin.
Selznick, Myron Archive. *File 169, Folder 3. The Harry Ransom Center.* Austin: University of Texas at Austin.
Spoto, Donald. *The Art of Alfred Hitchcock: Fifty Years of His Motion Pictures.* New York: Anchor Books, 1976.
Spoto, Donald. *The Dark Side of Genius: The Life of Alfred Hitchcock.* New York: Da Capo Press, 1999.
Spoto, Donald. *Spellbound by Beauty: Alfred Hitchcock and His Leading Ladies.* New York: Harmony Books, 2009.
Staiger, Janet. "Creating the Brand: Hitchcock's Touch." In *The Cambridge Companion to Alfred Hitchcock*, edited by Jonathan Freeman, 40–57. New York: Cambridge University Press, 2015.
Stam, Robert and Roberta Pearson. "Hitchcock's *Rear Window*: Reflexivity and the Critique of Voyeurism." *Enclitic* 7, no. 1 (Spring, 1983): 136–45.
Sterritt, David. *The Films of Alfred Hitchcock.* Boston: Cambridge University Press, 1993.
Stevens, Wallace. "Sunday Morning." In *The Collected Poems of Wallace Stevens*, edited by Chris Beyers, 71–75. New York: Vintage, 1990.
Taylor, John Russell. *Hitch: The Life and Times of Alfred Hitchcock.* New York: Da Capo Press, 1996.
Truffaut, Francois, ed. *Hitchcock/Truffaut.* New York: Simon & Schuster, 1983.
Walker, Michael. *Hitchcock's Motifs.* Amsterdam: Amsterdam University Press, 2005.
Weldon, Huw. Interviewer. *Monitor.* BBC. July 5, 1964.
Wood, Robin. *Hitchcock's Films.* Lancaster: Gazelle Books, 1978.
Wood, Robin. *Hitchcock's Films Revisited.* New York: Columbia University Press, 1989.
Zizek, Slavoj, ed. *Everything You Always Wanted to Know About Lacan (But Were Afraid to Ask Hitchcock).* London: Verso Books, 2010.

Index